159

HalfStraight

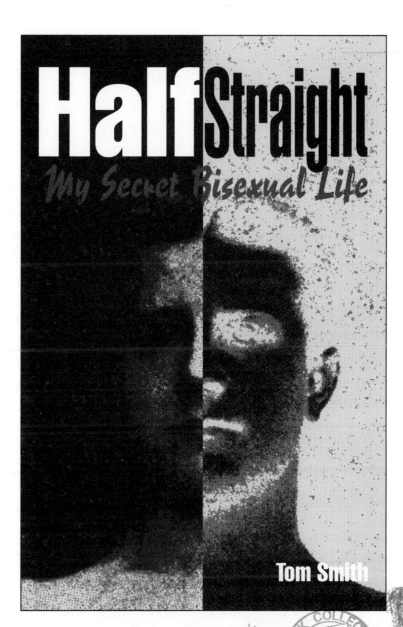

Half Straight

My Secret Bisexual Life

Tom Smith

Prometheus Books · Buffalo, New York

Published 1992 by Prometheus Books

96 95 94 93 92   5 4 3 2 1

Library of Congress Cataloging-in-Publication Data

Smith, Tom, 1924–
    Half straight : my secret bisexual life / by Tom Smith.
        p.   cm.
    ISBN 0-087975-734-5
    1. Bisexuality—United States—Case studies. 2. Smith, Tom,
1924–   . 3. Executives—United States—Biography. I. Title.
HQ74.S65   1992
306.76′5—dc20   92-3081
                                                                      CIP

Printed on acid-free paper in the United States of America

TO

My dear wife and
beloved son and daughter,
each of whom may never know
I wrote this book.

God loves them and so do I.

Contents

	Foreword by Vern L. Bullough	9
	Preface	13
1	How It All Started—Its Impact on Many Lives	15
2	Recognizing Reality and My Involvement	33
3	Some Early Experiences	47
4	Science Peers into the Closet and Gay Liberation Begins	65
5	Family Life as Husband and Father	75
6	Role of the Gay in Everyday Life	91
7	More Personal Experiences	103
8	Catastrophe Strikes the Gay World and Me Personally	121
9	God and Religion—The Homosexual Dilemma	141
10	A Look Back—Some Regrets	157
	Epilogue	169

Foreword

This book deals with bisexuality, the concept that an individual may be attracted to members of one's own sex as well as the opposite sex and be able to consummate sexual performance with both. The concept has a long history in mythology, but there are also some real historical examples: among the ancient Greeks, for instance, an adolescent boy was expected to have an adult male lover. Knowledge of this ancient practice may have influenced the work of Sigmund Freud who held that individual development included a homoerotic gang phase, although he felt most mature individuals eventually developed into heterosexuality. Alfred Kinsey argued that the three alternatives of heterosexuality, bisexuality, and homosexuality were much too rigid and put sexual preference on a seven point scale: exclusive heterosexuals were at one end and exclusive homosexuals at the other, with a wide middle ground for people who might be called bisexuals.

We know, for example, that there are what might be called situational homosexuals, really bisexuals, who while in prison or in other places where members of the opposite sex are not present turn to members of their own sex for pleasure. We also know that there is bisexuality among many of the higher animals.

Still, many of us, including myself, for long denied the existence of bisexuality. Situational bisexuality yes, but if an individual had a choice, he would be either homosexual or heterosexual. In this view, most bisexuals were really homosexuals who had to conform outwardly to societal norms by pretending to be heterosexual. Early evidence of bisexual behavior was also interpreted as experiments by the young or attempts of homosexuals to become heterosexuals.

Increasingly, however, there has been a willingness by many (myself included) to recognize the possibility that some people might well be bisexual, and even that bisexuality is fairly widespread and is not necessarily disguised homosexuality or heterosexuality. In 1975, Julius Fast and Hal Wells presented case studies of individuals who had sexual relations with both the opposite and the same sex and found both satisfying for different reasons. In 1978, Fred Klein went further, arguing that there are people who are basically bisexual. In fact he went so far as to hold that there is probably a basic capacity in all of us to respond erotically and emotionally/romantically to persons of either sex or gender, either simultaneously or serially. According to Klein, the response to each sex is not necessarily equal, but for a bisexual the response to both sexes is strong enough that such a person cannot fully identify as either a homosexual or heterosexual. They would be a three on the Kinsey scale, midway between 0 and 6, the two extremes. By 1987, Ivan Hill could report that 66 percent of the psychiatrists and 82 percent of the sex therapists surveyed by the Opinion Research Corporation of Princeton, N.J., regarded bisexuality as a bona fide classification, even though there was not always agreement among them on what was meant by bisexuality. They also disagreed on how many people might be classified as bisexual with estimates for this category ranging from 10 to 20 percent of the population. Estimates are guesswork, however, since most individuals engaged in a bisexual lifestyle do not go to psychiatrists or even to sex therapists. Many undoubtedly live their double lives in much the same way as the pseudonymous Tom Smith, the author of *Half Straight.*

Probably, most individuals who have a bisexual lifestyle have a definite preference for one sex or the other, and in view of the still-stigmatized social status of homosexuality, most probably adopt a heterosexual stance. This is easier at some stages of life than others. As individuals age, there often is a kind of funnel effect: they narrow their focus and concentrate more and more exclusively on one sex or the other. There is, however, still a lot that we do not know about such individuals. What is needed before we can come up with definitive answers is many more studies of individuals who have engaged in widespread bisexual activity.

This is why Tom Smith's autobiography is valuable. He is helping us chart the unexplored minefield that one must explore before coming up with any real answers to the question of bisexuality. Smith's original manuscript has gone through several revisions, as I have tried to get him to respond to basic questions which might be raised about his lifestyle. This has entailed the asking of basic questions about himself. In the process of trying to answer these questions, I think he has made a valuable contribution to the study not only of human sexuality but of what being human is all about. Few of us are willing to expose ourselves to quite the probing from an editor that he has undergone. The result, however, is a better understanding for me, at least, of the human psyche. Although Tom, perhaps as a result of the funnel effect, now says that he is a gay who finds it difficult to differentiate between heterosexual and homosexual sex, he hopes that his life will be perceived as a cultural revelation rather than a self-justifying exposé of a double life. So do I.

VERN L. BULLOUGH, Ph.D.
Series Editor
New Concepts in Human Sexuality

References

Fast, Julius, and Hal Wells. *Bisexual Living*. New York: A. M. Evans, 1975.

Hill, Ivan, ed. *The Bisexual Spouse*. New York: Barlina Books, 1987.

Klein, Fred. *The BiSexual Option*. New York: Arbor House, 1978.

Klein, Fritz, and Timothy Wolf, eds. *Bisexuality: Theory and Research*. New York: Harrington Park Press, 1985.

Rado, Sandor. "A Critical Examination of the Concept of Bisexuality." *Psychoanalytic Medicine* 2 (1940): 459–67.

Preface

I was married and the father of two children when I came to
the full realization that I am bisexual. For nearly forty years
I have led a secret double life. Although stimulating at times,
much of my life has been plagued by punishing guilt and an
all-consuming frustration. None of my immediate family, relatives, or life-long friends have any knowledge or even suspicion of my bisexuality and the experiences told of in the pages
ahead.

Writing this autobiography became an obsession. I had to
let the world know what bisexuality has done to me. But I was
not interested in writing just another shocking exposé of the
unconventional sex habits in the gay community, or a lurid diary
of obscenity and porn rhetoric. Rather it is my hope that this
book will be perceived by many not as a self-incriminating
disclosure but rather as a cultural revelation. There are many
others who like me appear to be the average, white, American,
male, business executive but in private are far from conventional. This is as much their story as it is mine.

The most common four-letter words will not be found in
this book. Nevertheless, to put some incidents in their true per-

spective, I have chosen to use certain characteristic and expressive expletives. These may be considered vulgar and offensive to some readers; if so, I offer my profound apologies.

I wouldn't do anything to embarrass, humiliate, or hurt my family. For this reason I have selected a fictitious pen name ("Tom Smith") for this book, in order to preserve and protect my identity. I have also altered a few names and dates; otherwise the ensuing pages tell it as it is and has been.

THE AUTHOR

1

How It All Started—
Its Impact on Many Lives

Whatever your attitude about homosexuality, there are individuals whom you greatly respect and admire, and in all probability you will never know that they are gay. Such a person might even be a loved one. Like straight people, gays are rich and poor, smart and dumb, handsome, beautiful, and ugly. They have been around as long as humans have inhabited the earth. These days, since it is no longer a crime to be homosexual, gays are being recognized for what they are. Many are among our most honored and distinguished intellectuals, professionals, artists, and corporate moguls.

And then there are people caught in the middle—half gay and half straight—like me, a devoted husband and father who is also gay. I am two psychologically confused, lonely people trapped in one restless body. My dual sexual personality has afflicted my life with an unrelenting anxiety that someday my secret will be exposed. This constant fear and the pressure of leading a secret double life has damaged my personality and affected my life physically, mentally, and spiritually. Why couldn't God have let me be just gay or straight, rather than both? It would have made life so much more tolerable.

In recent years I have realized that my emotions have had a striking effect on the psyches of my son and daughter. The thought of sexual exploitation with them never entered my mind. As a matter of fact, my apprehension about my bisexuality produced the opposite behavior. Now, as adults they think I had no feeling for them. They believe that I was insensitive to their emotional needs during their childhood years, and that I should have been more physical in showing my affection. Both of them individually feel this way. They probably have every right to have these feelings because for thirty to thirty-five years I have kept my guard up. For me love, emotion, affection, and sex were all intermingled into one entity, and knowing this, I developed a hands-off disposition with the ones I so dearly love. It's really sad.

For some strange reason it strikes me as awkward and tactless to show outward affection for my family, the ones I truly love. My attitude toward my wife is the same. I know my displays of affection for her are lackluster, and yet she is the only love of my life. For many years my wife has had no interest in sex; at times I have almost considered her to be asexual. Nevertheless, she is a very affectionate, caring person.

I have lived in a hard shell for most of my adult life. It developed sometime as a young adult when I became aware of my dual sexual nature. The realization produced a befuddling mental confusion and I constantly wondered whether there was something wrong with me. Was I really different? I tried to put it out of my mind, but it was always there. I felt whatever the answer was I had to hide it and soon it became a compulsion for me to conceal my emotions.

I have never had a serious gay relationship. I don't believe I could ever cohabitate with another man; it's just one of the many psychological complexities of my bisexuality.

At times I honestly don't know what I am and feel like a rudderless boat that will drift ashore wherever the winds will take me and this in spite of the fact I must be in control of every situation. I've been a man on the run with a chip on his shoulder trying to escape himself and the reality of his psychobiology. I have lived more lives than the proverbial cat and have the hide of an alligator and soul of a butterfly. In addition to mental agony and despair, bisexuality has left me suspended in time and space. I really want to be on both sides of the spectrum, but know I can't truthfully admit that to anyone without risking the loss of the loving family relationship with my wife, son, daughter, son-in-law, sisters, and now my grandkids, all of whom mean so much to me. I know my miserable temperament has left psychological scars on my wife, son, and daughter, even though I've tried so hard to be a good husband and loving respected father. Unknowingly, my bisexuality has had its impact on many lives.

Although I believe in God, I don't believe He is planning to "get even" with me for my sexuality here on earth. Society, not God, has laid the burden of guilt and transgression on me. Many of the problems in the world today are the outcome of the social controls and standards under which we live. This includes the very struggle for survival. It was only about twenty-five years ago that blacks began to realize that their problem was not a genetic one, but rather a social one. When that realization hit home, blacks discovered a place for themselves in God's plan. From then on, they were never the same again, because they were motivated in the direction of acceptance and achievement. I too know now that there is a place in God's plan for me.

Sixty-five years ago I was born in a medium-sized town in the great Central Valley of California. When I was only seven, my father died in an automobile accident. I have four sisters, two older and two younger. I was the only boy. Even though the country was recovering from the world's worst depression, my proud, courageous, young mother made a steadfast decision; she would raise her family alone without any outside help. With practically nothing to go on and in spite of the odds, she did just that. She was a resolute, religious woman imbued in her Catholic faith. She believed in miracles and her decision evolved into a big one. There was never another man in her life, so I didn't have a stepfather.

As I was growing up, there were no luxuries, but we never lacked any of the essentials. Our home was modest but it had lots of love and affection. My greatest deprivation was a father, a man to guide me and lean on. However, I didn't seem to realize it at the time, and whether or not having a dad would have had any bearing on my outcome, I just don't know. I somehow feel it wouldn't have made all that much difference, except for some fond memories. Not having a father created a serious sense of responsibility in me. Perhaps it even developed my exemplary conscientious character, which I may not have had otherwise. Certainly, it helped me to become a self-made man.

My first year of high school was spent in the minor seminary of a religious order. I had thoughts of becoming a priest, but after a couple of months in the seminary, my attitude changed greatly. Even at that tender age, in the months I was there, I did some serious soul searching and contemplated my future. I was very close to my family and family life meant so very much to me. I felt that I might want to be a father (not just the father of a flock of faithful). Perhaps this inclination and my feelings about family life were the result of growing up without a dad. Then, too, there were other influencing factors— order priests lead a much more rigid, regimented life than parish priests. When I left the seminary, my mother was happy to have me back home, but I also detected some disappointment. I think perhaps she may have thought if her only son was a priest, it could be her express ticket to heaven. God love her and rest her soul.

In high school I was attracted to the girls and the girls to me. Obviously, I was not a pansy and there was no lace on my shorts. I was popular with the guys too and involved in many activities—sports and academic. At home, religion was a part of our daily life and I had a solemn sense of moral awareness. At that age, sex was of little concern to me. The truth is, I hardly knew what it was all about and didn't take a lot of time to dwell on it. I realize now I missed so much of the good life in my early years. I had a fun personality and the only thing that ever got me into trouble was my uncontrollable sense of humor.

I was a spirited kid in high school. In my junior year, five or six of my buddies and I would occasionally skip afternoon classes on hot summer days to go skinny-dipping in the mighty high-water river nearby. We always went to the same secluded sandy beach where we could swim in the raw. There was usually lots of horseplay and body contact, but never any indication of sexual inclinations. I remember that two of the guys were extremely well endowed like me. But I was just a little different. Since I hadn't been circumcised, I was the only one in the group who had a foreskin. The guys would give me a relentless ribbing, calling me such things as "limpy" and "skin head." Possibly none of us were aware of or concerned about homosexuality at that time in our lives. I can decisively say I was not bisexual then. If there was a queer in the group, only God knew. We were all fun loving, red-blooded Americans. One of the boys went into the Marine Corps and was killed three years later on Iwo Jima.

One of those guys turned out to be my very best life-long friend—the brother I never had. He's a prosperous businessman now and straight as an arrow. We're extremely close, and his wife and my wife are very dear friends also. We've all known one another since high school. Here it is forty-five years later and none of them, including my wife, know I'm gay. We have had some wonderful times together, but never anything of a sexual nature.

The last summer I was in high school I worked as a "call boy." No, it's not what you're thinking. Call boys or crew callers were young men employed by Southern Pacific Railroad. Our responsibility was to wake up engineers, conductors, brakemen, and flagmen who were due for departure on late night or early morning freight and passenger trains. The crew member had to sign a call log verifying the exact time the caller made personal contact. We worked out of the dispatcher's office at the round-house and rode company-owned bicycles to the homes, residence hotels, boarding houses, and apartments of train crews who were required to live within very close proximity of the rail yards and depot. The bicycles were painted company colors, orange and black, and had a large SP logo on them. You could spot the bikes a block away.

One sultry summer night, shortly after 2 A.M., I went to the apartment of a single passenger conductor who was probably about forty to fifty years old. When he answered the door, he was standing there with a towel wrapped around his middle and invited me in. He told me he'd been up for an hour, had just finished showering and shaving, and was waiting for me. I only had two members of his crew to call and he was the second, so I accepted his invitation to come in. I had called on him once before. He asked if I would like to have a Coke and that sounded pretty good, because for me the middle of the night was like the middle of the day.

I was sitting in a chair sipping my Coke when he walked to within two feet of me and pulled off the towel. His penis was expanding and starting to stick out. But just at that point a telephone on a nearby table rang. It was the dispatcher telling him there had been a last minute development concerning his run and he needed to come in a half hour early for special instructions. When he hung up he was frustrated and disconcerted. He told me he had to get dressed and go over to the dispatch office; something had come up about his run. I thanked him for the Coke and left. I was so naive and unworldly I didn't perceive the implications. At that time in my young life I thought there was only male-female sex.

A few months later, after my summer job had terminated, an article appeared in the newspaper about my conductor acquaintance. He had been arrested on suspicion of sexual assault on a minor male crew caller. I never did find out the outcome of the case, if indeed there was a case. A couple of years later I realized that my brief encounter with him could have developed into my first experience with a homosexual.

Early in World War II my patriotism got the best of me and I left high school to join the navy. It had become difficult to concentrate on academic pursuits and plan for the future with the whole world in such chaotic turmoil.

In mid 1942, I had a weekend pass and was hitchhiking home from navy bootcamp in San Diego. During the war years, it was common to see servicemen hitchhiking on the highways and roads of the country. There were no freeways or expressways then, and it was considered downright patriotic for travelers to pick up men in uniform. Neither traveler nor hitchhiker had any reservations about it. My first ride let me out on Sepulveda Boulevard near Wilshire Boulevard in west Los Angeles. Sepulveda was a major highway then and the Westwood section, where I was waiting for my next ride, was lined on both sides with high eucalyptus trees. It was shaded and very picturesque bordering on a large veterans national cemetery and a section of the beautiful UCLA campus. It's one of the most affluent areas in Southern California, near Beverly Hills and Bel Air.

I was standing by the side of the road, in my navy uniform, when a cute little yellow MG, with the top down, pulled up. The driver, a man wearing dark sunglasses, leaned over and opened the door for me. After I got in, he took off his sunglasses, and I stared in amazement at a famous movie star of that era. He was a handsome character actor and at that time was probably about fifty years old. I was eighteen and, when I now look at photos of myself at that point in life, I realize I was a tender, baby-faced kid. He wanted to know where I was going and how soon I had to be there. He said he had something I'd be interested in seeing and it was nearby. It was early Friday afternoon, I had a three-day liberty pass, and was only about three hours from home. Being spellbound by the presence of this screen star, I agreed to go along.

My new ride drove into a sidestreet motel in Westwood Village. When approaching the motel, he put his dark glasses back on. He was already registered and may have had someone register for him. When we got into his room, he dropped his pants and there it was. Now I was in a different kind of shock and was unable to register any emotion. The next thing I knew, he was unbuttoning the thirteen buttons on the flap of my seaman's pants. When he touched my penis there was a vibrant reaction and in seconds I had a stiff erection. He had taken his pants off and now he stripped off the rest of his clothes. Then, he pulled down my pants, took off my shoes, and removed my shorts. He reached for a jar of Vaseline on the dresser, unscrewed the cap, and began rubbing some on my penis. By this point, my bewilderment had turned to fright and I said, "What do you think you're doing?" My new acquaintance said, "I want you to stick that gorgeous thing in me." I said, "No, I don't think so."

Then, with his big penis in his hand, Mr. Celebrity asked me to lie down on the bed. I said, "What for?" He said, "Maybe you'd prefer this." I don't recall exactly what I said, but it meant unequivocally "no way." He tried to tell me that it's a beautiful experience and that maybe I was just not used to it. I said, "I think you've got the wrong guy." But the next thing I knew, he had dropped to his knees in front of me and was oral copulating. After a couple of minutes, I had an orgasm in his mouth. I was in a state of total confusion—there was something good about it and yet, at the same time, something awful. I realize now the awfulness was my religious upbringing showing through and creating a guilty conscience. I couldn't respond and wouldn't touch him. I think he sensed I was scared, so he didn't push for anything more after my orgasm. I'm sure he thought he had a real "hayseed" from the boondocks of Iowa. In fact, I was a real hayseed, but from central California.

We were in his room less than twenty minutes. When we were ready to leave, he offered me a ten dollar bill. I didn't want to take it, but he insisted. Ten dollars was a lot of money in those days and even more so for a serviceman. That was the only time in my entire life I have taken money for a sexual favor, and that favor was given in a state of coercion. He drove me back to where he had picked me up, about ten minutes away. There were several other servicemen hitchhiking in that area, and I have often wondered how many other young men he may have taken to that motel room that day.

This was my first encounter with a homosexual and a most unusual one because of the personality involved. I was a very impressionable and vulnerable country boy. As I think about it now, the reason I was cooperative to any degree may have been that I considered myself lucky to have been selected by this famous guy. He was very well hung and extremely proud of it. If I had been more mature, I could have had the time of my life. However, the whole thing was simply repulsive to me. He had wanted to kiss me, but that I wouldn't let him do, regardless of the personality involved. I'm sure he expected much more participation and cooperation on my part, and I must have been a great disappointment to him.

In later years, when I thought about that episode, it reminded me of an attempted rape of a young girl by an older man. If an officer of the law had apprehended my celebrity acquaintance in the course of the encounter, he would undoubtedly have been charged with statutory rape. Since I was a minor male, rather than a female, the judicial system at that point in time would have come down mercilessly hard on him. He most likely would have been sentenced to a state prison and in view of my military status, it could even have been a federal penitentiary. In deference to any living relatives, I will not make known the actor's name here. It was not a headline moniker, but does appear in Kitty Kelly's book *Nancy Reagan*.

I have never told a straight person about this, so I guess it's time I should let the world know. This incident was my virgin initiation into homosexual and bisexual activities. Could it have been the catalyst that eventually caused me to become bisexual; who knows? It undoubtedly triggered the beginning of my sexual idiosyncrasies and the unfolding of a passion for sex in deviating forms. I don't believe in the theory that our genes, at the time of conception, will determine whether we will be heterosexual or homosexual. And, certainly, I don't believe our sexual preferences are hereditary. As far as I'm concerned, sexual preferences are as simple as dessert preferences: some people like ice cream, but don't like candy; others like candy, but don't like ice cream. And some like both. Whatever your preference, as the bumper sticker says, "Eat dessert first— life is so uncertain."

Another important incident in my coming of age occurred in 1943 on a Saturday afternoon in the East Bay Terminal Building in San Francisco. I was on the lower level and noticed a group of people in the doorway of the men's room. I looked through the doorway and to my amazement saw three police officers talking to a sailor and Mr. Brady, my high school geometry teacher. I was in Brady's classroom less than a year before. There were lots of sailors around, other than myself, so I asked one what was going on. He said the old guy was giving the "swabby" a "blow job" in one of the toilet stalls when a plainclothes police officer came in to check out the place. Brady was not an old man, probably about forty-five to fifty, but when I was still a teenager, it seemed pretty old.

San Francisco was only about a four and a half hour drive from my hometown in the valley. Mr. Brady had been one of my most admired and respected high school teachers. I absolutely couldn't believe this. I just knew he couldn't be "queer." He was a family man and often talked about his family in classroom discussions. His wife was also a teacher, in an elementary school. In a short time, a large crowd had gathered and Brady never saw me in the sea of faces. It was obvious he was humiliated and mortified. At one point I had an urge to step forward and tell the officers I knew this man and he couldn't possibly have done that. But something told me that might not be the prudent thing to do.

I watched as the officers led Brady and the sailor out of the building to a police car and drove away. My ship sailed the next day and I was to be gone for an indefinite period of time, which turned out to be two months. I have often wondered what happened to Brady. He probably lost his job, tenure, and his family, and was blackballed from getting another teaching job for the rest of his income-earning life. That is ruination. Only God knows whether or not what he did was right or wrong. He was satisfying the needs and desires of another person as well as himself. Certainly, it wasn't the right time or place and he obviously showed poor judgment.

Another of my navy hitchhiking experiences took place on a beautiful early afternoon in the spring of 1943 in Oakland, California. I had a three-day liberty pass and had taken a bus

from Treasure Island in San Francisco Bay to Oakland. I was
on my way home to the San Joaquin Valley. After disembark-
ing from the bus, I walked about three blocks to a more favor-
able spot for hitchhiking.

I had been standing at the curb for about ten minutes when
this impressive (at least to me at that time) automobile pulled
up to offer me a ride. I think it was a late model Buick or
Oldsmobile. The driver motioned for me to get in. He had the
air of a charming, gracious businessman and was dressed like
a San Francisco Montgomery Street broker: three-piece pinstripe
suit and hat on the front seat. As I opened the car door to get
in, he put his hat on the back seat.

My philanthropic driver was going to San Leandro, not far
from where I was heading. He said he knew a short cut through
the Oakland hills, and after we had been driving about fifteen
or twenty minutes, we came to a section of the road that was
tree-lined and wooded on each side. He reached under his seat
and pulled out a manila envelope and told me there were some
pictures inside I might enjoy looking at. When I pulled out the
photos I couldn't believe what I was seeing. At that time, since
I was still a pretty naive kid, there could only be one way to
describe it—electrifying pornography.

My benefactor pulled off the highway onto a little side road
in a wooded area. At that point I had an uncontained erection straining against the thirteen buttons of my navy seaman's
pants. As I was unconsciously scrutinizing the photos, the man
began opening the buttons on the flap of my pants. Before I
really knew what was happening, he had pulled down my shorts
and had my penis in his mouth. My first reaction was one of
repulsion. As I look back now, I feel very certain that my religious guilt would not allow me to savor the ecstasy of the
moment. My acquaintance had opened his pants and took my
hand and put it on his penis and testicles. I couldn't respond
to that, but did soon have an orgasm in his mouth. After we

were finished he gave me some Kleenex to clean myself up, and soon we were on our way. A short time later, he dropped me off alongside the highway in San Leandro. I was totally confounded, and little did I know what had just happened was an occult manifestation that would have a profound effect on my entire life in the years ahead.

In my middle and late teens, the fact that I had not been circumcised became a source of inhibition and embarrassment to me. My foreskin hung down about a half inch over the head of my penis. Even in high school, in the gym showers it was obvious I was different. I sort of felt like a freak.

When I went into navy bootcamp in 1942, I felt even more ill at ease because I was thrown together with so many guys. You just didn't very often see a guy in the showers with a foreskin, perhaps one in fifteen or twenty. Sometimes, I'd catch a guy staring at me, and I'd have to turn the other way. I dreaded our weekly venereal-disease examinations, known as "short arm inspections." Sixty sailors had to stand nude in front of their bunks in our large dorm-like room in the barracks building. There were fifteen double bunks on either side of a wide aisle. A medical officer (doctor), along with a hospital corpsman, came down the aisle to inspect the genitals of each sailor. The corpsman had a flashlight and was looking for body lice (crabs) in the pubic hair. As they approached each sailor, one would shout, "Skin it back and milk it down." This meant, pull your foreskin back and squeeze your penis. If you had an infection and there was any pus in your urethral tract, it would ooze out of the head of your penis. There were always four or five guys who had to step aside for further examination and treatment. "Short arm inspection" was always an embarrassment to me. Invariably the doctor would say, "Pull it back further, all the way, sailor."

In 1944, I was wounded in the South Pacific and recuperated in a field hospital on the tropical island of Samoa for several weeks. During that time, I talked one of the surgeons into circumcising me. He was about fifty years old and knew precisely what he was doing; he didn't take too much off or leave too much.

In my ward were two marines confined to beds on either side of me. The day after my circumcision they plotted a little conspiracy. They were curious to see what would happen if I had an erection during the healing process; so they began telling dirty stories back and forth across my bed. Within a few minutes my penis was standing straight up. Thirty minutes later the dressing was drenched in blood—I had busted my stitches and had to be taken back to surgery. My marine buddies satisfied their curiosity and got their kicks. After that, I got very attentive, loving care from a gracious hospital corpsman, who delighted in changing my dressings. He was probably queer.

In retrospect, I have long realized that circumcision was a big mistake; however, then I wanted to conform. Men who have not been circumcised are much more sensitive and passionate during sex and get much more enjoyment out of it than those who have been circumcised. That has been my experience and observation with men I have known who have an uncut penis. Now I know I left some of the best of me in the South Pacific.

The United States is one of just a few countries where circumcision is a common practice. 4,100 American male babies are circumcised every day. As a result, an estimated 200 suffer what skilled surgeons call "excessive penile loss." However, many doctors now are discouraging parents of new-born males from having the procedure done. A trend is rapidly developing not to circumcise. Perhaps in the next 20 or 30 years, the guy in the showers and locker room who is circumcised will be the oddball.

While still in the navy, I came home and married my high school sweetheart. I will call her Sue. Even though I was now a man of the world, Sue was still my choice and has remained my choice for more than forty years. By this time I had been involved in the homosexual encounters described above. Both incidents had been repulsive and even offensive to me. I didn't have the slightest idea that I had any homosexual tendencies.

In the early months of our marriage, Sue and I had an apartment in San Francisco. My ship was based there and I would be in every few weeks for a week or ten days at a time, with the exception of when I was wounded and was in the navy mobile hospital on the island in the South Pacific for two months. In spite of the fact that there was a global war raging, we would have some fun times when I was in port on short-term leaves. I had heard so much about the place, that one time I took Sue to Finocchio's on Broadway in the North Beach area of San Francisco. Finocchio's was a notorious night club and boasted that it had the world's greatest female impersonators. It was one of the most celebrated night spots in the city. The night Sue and I were there, a rotund, older gay who was impersonating Sophie Tucker was the "mistress of ceremonies" for the show. We had a table in front of the stage, and the stage lights were so bright that I had put my hand over my forehead. It must have looked like my thumb was in my mouth because at one point "Sophie" looked down at me and said, "Get your thumb out of your mouth, sonny; that's the way I got my start." Sitting there in my navy uniform, I was downright embarrassed. On the way home, Sue asked me whether I thought that guy or that "it" thought I might be a budding homosexual. I dismissed the suggestion with, "Don't be ridiculous." She said, "I'm only kidding, but you did add a little spice to his routine."

Today, Finocchio's is still in existence and can now boast of fifty years of the world's greatest female impersonators. It is truly a San Francisco institution. I know of two young men in the show today who proudly admit that their fathers were in the Finocchio chorus line twenty-three and twenty-seven years

ago. So, what does that tell you? All gay people are not homosexual. There are lots of bisexuals, who enjoy the best of two
worlds.

At the end of the war, in the late summer of 1945, I was
discharged from the navy. Sue quit her job in San Francisco
and we returned to our hometown in the central valley. I had
come home to be reeducated and to change the world. Sue
and I had been married just a year before and she was now
expecting our first child. Three months later our beautiful
daughter arrived. I will call her Margie. The devil-may-care days
were now gone. I was a husband and father and had a family
to support. The adjustment was a difficult, demanding process.
However, I managed to get on track and keep family and
marriage together.

For a number of years I was physically and mentally lost.
There was something haywire with my life. In spite of my lack
of a formal education, I had a knack for landing competitive,
above-average jobs and even junior-executive positions. But there
was always something wrong, a restlessness that wouldn't let
my potential materialize. I was never satisfied, it was difficult
to concentrate on the job at hand, and I was always on the
move, living in the unsatisfactory present and oblivious of the
future. My priorities were out of whack and I couldn't find my
purpose in life.

Up to that point, I had considered myself a "straight arrow."
A few months later, I began having some doubts when I found
myself reminiscing over the male sexual encounters in which
I had been involved while in the navy. I believe this is where
the real frustration set in. At the same time I was beginning
to have a bisexual urge, Sue's sexual enjoyment and desire were
waning and have never been the same. Perhaps the rigors of
motherhood were taking their toll on her own sexual pleasures.
This became a very difficult and perplexing time in my life.
I was torn between two directions and at the same time knew

I had made a life-long commitment of fidelity to just one of those directions. Soon my character and demeanor began to show strains of discontent—discontent that as the years passed turned into diminished love and a mean temper. It was the time in my life I should have faced up to my dilemma, but I just didn't have the guts. I couldn't cope with making that decision.

2

Recognizing Reality
and My Involvement

When I unquestionably knew I was gay, the die had long been cast—I was a husband and father and very much involved in family life. We lived in a smart, fashionable section of San Francisco. At age thirty-seven I was a senior executive in a major East Bay transportation and industrialization organization. For further reference, I will call it the XYZ Group. My daughter was now sixteen, my son was eleven, and my wife a year younger than I. Ten or twelve years prior to that time, I had an occasional homosexual encounter, but was not leading an unrestrained gay lifestyle. Now I had become more uninhibited about my bisexuality, yet I still very much loved my wife and daughter and son.

I just can't be sure whether or not I would have become gay if I had been getting all the sex I wanted from my wife. They say the only reason men cheat on their wives is because they're not getting enough at home. I'm not so sure about that. If Sue were a highly sexed woman, I wonder what my sexual orientation would be today? So much for the fantasy thinking.

In any case, I felt the need to go outside of my marriage to satisfy my sexual urges. Whether I turned to gay sex because of my early experiences in the navy or because gay sex was so easy and available in San Francisco, I just don't know.

Homosexuality was certainly not condoned or tolerated in social circles or the work force. Nevertheless, San Francisco seemed to be the homosexual capital of the entire country. At that time there were nine public homosexual bathhouses in the city, often referred to as Turkish Baths. I had been told there were a couple private clubs for gays, but never pursued that possibility. There were also numerous gay bars, but they didn't offer the immediate convenience and possibilities of the baths. If you did go to a gay bar and met a guy you were attracted to, if he couldn't take you home and you couldn't take him home, you'd wind up going to one of the baths anyway. I was not a service club joiner, such as Rotary, Exchange, Kiwanis, Lions, etc. Perhaps if I had been, it would have expanded my male sexual contacts. There are undoubtedly gentlemen in those organizations who are interested in gay relationships. But because of my family status and self-imposed secrecy, the gay baths were my best outlet and source for making contacts. As a result, in those days I embarked upon a long, long association with the gay baths.

The gay baths were and still are, where they exist, a meeting place and rendezvous for homosexuals and bisexuals; they provided a great environment for impersonal sex. The small rooms were really cubicles, each with a small built-in bed. Most had a shelf on the wall or a bedside stand and hooks for hanging clothes on hangers. Some even had a full-length mirror at one end of the bed or even on the ceiling and usually a light with dimmer switch. These rooms had one and only one purpose —sex. Depending on the size of the bathhouse, there may have been anywhere from thirty to sixty or more single rooms. Some had communal rooms with from two to six beds. Most baths also contained orgy rooms; in some there were even two or three. These dimly lighted rooms contained pads anywhere from ten to twelve or fourteen feet in diameter. I have seen multiple orgies on the pads with as many as ten to fourteen guys in action. A few years ago in San Francisco, one of the popular baths was in an old downtown converted warehouse building. The orgy area was a large upstairs loft with deep-pile carpets. It was absolute pandemonium on Friday and Saturday nights.

In most baths, when a guy came in, it was very much like checking into a motel or hotel. He would sign in (usually with a fictitious name), pay the tab (between $7 and $10), and be given a room key and two towels. One towel was referred to as a wrapper. He could check his wallet and other valuables into a secured lock box. After disrobing in his room, a guy usually wrapped the towel around his middle before leaving the room to cruise the corridors of the bathhouse.

The common practice in the baths was either to cruise the halls or stay in your room with the door open and size up those who were cruising. If you stayed in your room with the door open, and you appealed to one of the cruisers, he might stick his head in the door and ask if he could come in. If he appealed to you, you simply invited him in and the scenario began. Many bathhouse customers had sex more than once in one afternoon or evening.

The baths had various facilities and accommodations depending on location and the clientele catered to. All baths had toilet and shower rooms and almost all of them had wet steam rooms; many also had dry saunas. Some even had bidet/enema fixtures. Other equipment and facilities that one commonly saw were exercise and workout rooms with sophisticated gym equipment, snack bars, massage rooms with full-time masseurs around the clock, small indoor swimming pools and spas (hot tubs and whirlpools), and in certain suburban areas, small outside gardens and outdoor swimming pools shielded with high solid fences or walls to assure seclusion and privacy. Here you could do "it" on the grass or at poolside. Most baths, in addition to having stereo music throughout, had a movie room, which was very much like an orgy room with a large-screen, closed-circuit television continually showing hard-core pornographic films. You could do your "thing" on deep-pile carpeting and at the same time watch porn flicks with your selected partner or partners. Some of the more luxurious bathhouses had a lounge area with one or more televisions and perhaps a pool table. Some even had, in addition to masseurs, manicure services, hair stylists, and valet services.

Most of the facilities in gay baths were used in the nude. The wrapper (wrap-around towel) was for the tender, timid guys when cruising the corridor and common areas. However, it was surprising to see how many guys used the wrapper. I suppose they wanted to leave something to the imagination of the other guys rather than stroll the hallways completely naked. Then, too, there were some baths that required you to wear the wrapper in the hallways and common areas. As a bisexual, I have often thought how great it would be if there were both men and women in the baths. That would truly be the best of two worlds.

Gay baths have been around for a long time. The Ellis Baths in San Francisco had been in existence for more than forty years when it was closed by the city health department in October 1984. It was situated on Ellis Street across from the San Francisco Hilton Hotel. When it opened, there was no Hilton and there was no connection between the word gay and homosexual; the customers were known as queers. Although in the heart of the city, the Ellis Street Baths had a small indoor swimming pool and the facilities were used in the nude. It was one of the nicer meeting places for homos and "bi"s in its day. It made the Hilton across the street a desirable and convenient stop for traveling gay business executives. I met many fine gentlemen there (all gentlemen don't prefer blondes). After its closing, the entrance to the Ellis Baths was boarded up for more than two years, in spite of the property's prime location. It seemed that the owners were waiting it out, hoping there would be an immediate, miraculous virus vaccine and cure for AIDS and that there would be a reemergence of the baths as a social enclave for gays.

Prior to the onset of AIDS, gay baths could be found in almost all major metropolitan cities in the United States. Reverend Jerry Falwell, leader of the Moral Majority, has referred to gay bathhouses as sites of "sub-animal behavior." The truth of the matter is, Falwell is right, but how could he be so positive unless he's been there? Credible people don't quote hearsay.

Black gay baths were becoming popular at about the time of the AIDS outbreak (1980–81). These were establishments that catered to a black clientele and trade, not that you wouldn't find blacks in almost all gay baths. When I was with the XYZ Group, I knew a gay black police sergeant in Oakland. It was his dream someday to own and operate a black gay bathhouse. I lost track of him some years ago and whether or not his dream materialized I do not know.

The baths, for many years, were a humane outlet for homosexuals. This was particularly true of a bisexual like myself with a wife and family at home—the guy who could not take advantage of gay social contacts in the evenings or on weekends through clubs and church groups. One time I heard a retired superior court judge tell a businessmen's luncheon that he favored regulated prostitution, such as exists in Nevada. It's big business in Las Vegas and Reno and produces substantial revenues for local jurisdictions in the state. The judge believed prostitution has a propitious, humanitarian place in society. It was his contention that it is a deterrent to rape. Perhaps the gay baths, in fulfilling a need, have also been a deterrent. In most major metropolitan cities, male prostitution is as big a headache to law enforcement officials as is female prostitution. It's a stark reality that Americans hand over $40 million every day to prostitutes and prostitution is an awesome revenue-producing business. If I were to pay for sex, I'd prefer to spend my money with a woman rather than a man. Sex comes so much easier with men.

A large percentage of gay men have an insatiable sexual drive. The baths used to be the place to let it all hang out and what you saw was what you got. Many times I have spent three or four hours in a gay bath and had sexual encounters with four or five different men, who were total strangers. In that period of time I may have had two to three orgasms and brought two or three other individuals to climax.

One time while in one of the popular San Francisco baths, I was approached by a little old man. He let me know immediately he couldn't ejaculate, but that he had some unique techniques and could teach me some new tricks. The old guy was clean, had a good smell and a certain charisma and magnetism, so I capitulated and invited him to my room. He told me he was 82 years old, but very young in spirit. He did, indeed, have some unique techniques. He removed his false teeth and his fellatio (oral copulation) produced a delirious, sensual thrill. When I had a climax in his mouth, I could feel his little wrinkled body quiver. My orgasm probably produced for him a fantasy orgasm. Obviously, he was living in the past. He was ecstatic about having incited me to come. I somehow felt I had been a philanthropist that day.

My little old playmate was wearing a "cock ring." So, what is a "cock ring"? It's a round metal ring that fits over the penis and testicles together and rests firmly against the body, causing an incessant pressure that induces an erection of the penis. Cock rings come in three or four sizes and are either silver plated or nickel plated. There are also "cock thongs." These miniature, adjustable, leather thongs produce the same result as the rings. Usually, the rings and thongs are very effective, depending on any chemical imbalance in the body (liquor, certain drugs, etc.) and advanced old age. Obviously, for my little 82-year-old acquaintance, a "cock ring" was a lost cause. They don't work in all cases and his was one. At any rate, he was trying, and coping with old age is sometimes a cruel experience.

The baths, at that time, were my only source for meeting and having sex with other gay men. I would usually patronize one of the baths each week in the afternoon, telling my secretary that I was going to be gone for three or four hours for an outside meeting or to keep an impromptu appointment. I'd come up with a slightly different version of the same story each day, and she never suspected. She was a sweet family lady with a devoted husband, son, and daughter. They were a very religious family and perhaps that ruled out any suspicion she might have had regarding my activities outside of the office. Religious people are sometimes tremendously naive. However, in the office she was a top-rated executive secretary and my right arm for ten years.

If moralists, other than Falwell, had the slightest idea of what went on in steam baths, they would label them wicked dens of iniquity. They might even characterize the patrons as depraved and perverted. But, what does all that mean? It means simply that people have different moral ideals and ethics, dissimilar and divergent religious and social mores. It doesn't mean they're criminals or mentally deranged. Let's face it—we have natural animal instincts. Should they be totally inhibited because of man-made mores? Many puritanical individuals believe sex is only for procreation. I thank God that they are in the minority, and I thank Him too for the animal proclivities that make life so stimulating.

Even though most of the gay baths throughout the country have been closed, there is one popular place where you can still let it all hang out—the YMCA. The world-wide organization with 2,045 local, autonomous clubs in the United States has more than 14,000,000 members coast to coast. The membership includes some of the most honorable and respected business and professional people of the community. Most of the local Ys have health and fitness club facilities with private sections for both men and women. The Y is not generally thought of as a meeting place for gays, but many clubs turn out to be that way. The atmosphere is conducive to men interested in men and women interested in women.

The Y that I belong to has a membership in excess of 1,100. The facilities in the men's private section—the locker room and showers, wet and dry saunas, and the immense spa—are used in the nude. The only things missing are the private rooms, which were the nucleus of the gay baths. If a guy appeals to you and you make eye-to-eye contact, there is a delicate balance in your glances that dictates the tone of conversation. If you are on the same wavelength, you may make arrangements to meet elsewhere. But, then, there is that curse hanging over your head—AIDS.

Theories About Sexual Preference

There are many, varying ideas about why and how men and women become homosexual and bisexual. The key determining factor in sexual preference has long puzzled sociologists, psychologists, biologists, and others in the scientific world. Freud espoused the theory that we are all born bisexual, and only later develop a preference. Similarly, Kinsey believed there are homosexual tendencies in all of us. Yet in my experience, a true, unadulterated male homosexual will have nothing whatsoever to do sexually with a woman. Men are the sole focus of his sexuality. This exclusive same-sex drive is usually true of most lesbians. However, the bisexual is truly a mixed bag, a combination of homosexual and heterosexual, and this is what makes the whole thing a rare phenomenon.

I just don't believe I was born bisexual. As I mentioned earlier, I became aware of my bisexuality first in my early twenties. It's possible that the sexual revolution of the '60s had an effect on me. Many young men, and some older, became homo or bi during this period. The bywords then were: "If it feels good, do it"; "Don't knock it if you haven't tried it"; and "Try it, you might like it." It just may be that the bywords got to me.

Personality also has a lot to do with sexual preference. I have always been a person motivated by change and diversion, and unable to tolerate monotony. So far, I have made three separate career changes and my life has been a process of continuous metamorphosis. As a young man working for the railroad, how could I have ever thought that later in life I would be writing a book on such disdainful subject matter? Perhaps all of my various personality characteristics and talents have had a bearing on my being bisexual.

The least reputable theory about homosexuality is that it's a disease. Of course, such a notion is ludicrous. Homosexuality is no more a disease than celibacy. If it were, the Catholic Church would be harboring hundreds of thousands of diseased priests, monks, nuns, and brothers around the world.

In my opinion, some heterosexuals who become bi or gay experience a kind of heterosexual burn-out and feel that it's time for something else. When life becomes boring, existence difficult, and the wonder and magic of being alive start to fade, why should anyone resist change? If we become trapped in a dull, lifeless rhythm, perhaps it's time to give up our resistance to lifestyle changes and dance to a new step. In my case, I have discovered that change is the greatest source of stimulation and continued growth.

Generally speaking, I think gays are resolute, indomitable

people. They have to roll with the punches, and, as a result, develop an inner toughness and strong will to survive. My own situation is a prime example. Years ago it became apparent that none of my loved ones were gay. So, I made the unyielding decision never to come out of the "closet." I chose to lead a double life not because I was chicken or afraid to face up to it, but because of the possible damaging effect such disclosure could have on my relationship with those who mean so much to me. Sometimes my life has been hell—torment, frustration, and remorseful guilt. Nevertheless, at other times it seems that the positive outweighs the negative. If I had been lacking in strength mentally, I would have blown my brains out long ago.

Gay Stereotypes

Often people try to stereotype gays. If a man is a bachelor and has no girlfriends, he is immediately suspect. If a man has certain soft and dainty characteristics, he too may be in doubt. That's pure hogwash. Some of the most effeminate men would never dream of touching another man or letting another man touch them. At the same time some of the most macho males are totally gay. Your next door neighbor or a business partner could be gay and you may never know. For that matter, you could have a gay father, son, or brother or a lesbian mother, daughter, or sister and never know. So what? What you don't know may be best for you. My wife, daughter, and son don't know. What effect knowing would have on our loving relationship remains to be seen and I don't want to risk that eventuality.

There are divergent characters and personalities in the gay world just as there are in the heterosexual world. By no means do all gays patronize steam baths and gay bars. There is a wide span of introverts and extroverts among gays, just as there is among straights. On the other hand, I do believe that many more homosexuals than heterosexuals are promiscuous. This is born out by in-depth research studies of innumerable sociologists and psychologists. Gays by their very sexual orientation are much less inhibited. Nonetheless, there are lots of reclusive gay people. They usually are harboring damaging and even ruinous feelings of guilt, shame, or disgrace. I know—I lived with that paradoxical complex for thirty years. In reality, such conflicted individuals are often persons of strong moral fiber and are very much committed to preserving their honor and integrity.

Aristotle described friendship as "one soul in two bodies." I believe this appropriately applies to gays. Homosexuals, particularly, have a common bond, almost an aura that is not perceived by most heterosexuals. Sadly enough, most heterosexuals will not attempt to comprehend homosexuality, let alone tolerate it; even if not openly hostile, they often internalize their homophobia. This is why the term "closet" has come into play in past years regarding homosexuality. Many gays fearing reprisals if it were commonly known they were homo or bi—loss of a job, family rejection, or other damaging torments—remained in the closet. Now gays are coming out of the closet in increasing numbers, due to a more tolerant attitude on the part of society as a whole.

Pornography: Another Outlet

When there isn't a guy or gal available and the anxiety and pressure rises to the exploding point, there is an alternative. It's not one of my first choices, but when the "steam has to blow," it's better than nothing. The source is the closed-circuit television viewing booths in adult bookstores. These show hard-core pornography, the type that are completely explicit and leave nothing to the imagination. In most stores, you put a quarter in the slot for three minutes of viewing. If you haven't had an orgasm after five or seven quarters, you weren't in such urgent, compelling need after all. I have spent umpteen dollars in these booths in various cities around the country. It's a messy situation, but I learned long ago to take along a pocket full of Kleenex or an oversized handkerchief.

I can't really remember the first time I masturbated. I don't know whether it was before or after I was married. It's inconceivable to think I did not masturbate somewhere in my middle or late teens. In any case, by the time I was twenty-five, masturbation played a big part in my life. When the tension and stress would build up to the breaking point, I would take an "old friend" in hand and let it all come out. But in recent years, masturbation just doesn't get the job done for me. Now I need fraternal, sympathetic, responsive stimulus, and this is where my bisexuality is such an advantage. It's easier to fornicate with guys than with gals, especially when you're married.

It's too bad one has to pay for pornographic stimulation to satisfy the need to masturbate. Factual statistics show that Americans spend nearly $10 million a day on pornography. At least a quarter of a million people a day, in this country alone, attend full-length adult movies. With the advent of the VCR, millions of Americans view hard-core heterosexual and homosexual pornography on their home televisions every day. Not so in my home. But I have been a participant in video-viewing orgies in the apartments, condominiums, and homes of a number of friends. Ten million dollars a day is a staggering sum for pornography, even though it covers a wide spectrum of merchandise and services (exclusive of prostitution), most of which comes from adult and gay bookstores and X-rated movie theaters.

Many communities and even metropolitan cities have attempted to close down adult bookstores but with little success, due to the legal ramifications involved. We are now living in an era of open expression and freedom of choice. If an individual wishes to buy a magazine that explicitly and graphically shows sex acts, according to the United States Supreme Court, he or she has a right to do so. The only adult and pornographic bookstores I have heard of being closed by municipalities were within sight of a school or church, and certainly this is understandable.

3

Some Early Experiences

On a Christmas Eve in the early 1960s, my wife and I had a hurtful argument. Now I can't even recall the cause of that violent verbal clash. I was drinking pretty heavily at the time and that may be what obliterated some of my memory. At any rate, sometime in the late evening Sue took our son and daughter and checked into a motel. The following morning, Christmas Day, I awoke and found them gone. I was devastated. We had never had such a traumatic family dispute before (and never have again since then), and at Christmas, of all times. I began calling friends, trying to learn, without causing suspicion, if Sue had been in touch with them. It was a futile effort.

We were to have dinner that day with some very dear friends and their daughter and son-in-law. They lived down the San Francisco Peninsula, about twenty-five minutes away in San Mateo. We usually had our own holiday dinners with family and relatives, but Sue wanted to take them up on their invitation that particular year. They had been our guests the year before. About 10:30 A.M. the phone rang. It was the female half of our friends. She said Sue had called her about 8 o'clock and told her we were all under the weather—looked like the flu and the kids were surprisingly ill with temperatures. She asked to speak to Sue, and in a moment of swift reaction, I told her Sue had decided on going to church by herself. Our friend said she was disappointed we wouldn't be with them that day, but understood the circumstances. She said to let Sue know she'd help any way she could. For me, it was a remorseful thought and I knew I was fully responsible for an ill-timed, needless calamity that would have damaging emotional effects on my wife and kids.

My wife is an impulsive person and not one to give in easily; so I figured she might not be back until evening or possibly even the next day, since the kids were out of school. I was "licking my wounds" and in mid-afternoon decided to go to my favorite steam bath. Most of the baths were open twenty-four hours a day, 365 days a year, but on Christmas Day I didn't think there would be anyone there at all. At least I would benefit from the relaxation of the steam, I said to myself, and after the night before, I needed this therapy. To my amazement, there were five or six handsome, interesting-appearing men in the place. I struck up an intriguing conversation with one of these gentlemen, and this initial meeting eventually developed into an intimate seven-year friendship. I will call him Chris. Chris was five years older than I, a handsome, blond, blue-eyed Adonis, about six feet tall. I was in the place four hours and in that time Chris and I "plundered" each other twice.

He was a civil engineer for one of the country's largest international industrial construction firms. At the time, he was project coordinator for a top-secret overseas military installation, which was a sensitive security position, so he was on standby status to be available for any situation on twenty-four-hour notice. Chris and his family lived in Menlo Park, about thirty-five minutes down the San Francisco Peninsula. About two years after I met him, quite by accident, I met his gorgeous, sexy wife in his office. I had also seen photos of his two kids, a son and a daughter.

They were a beautiful all-American family.

On this particular day (Christmas), Chris was also feeling sorry for himself, and perhaps that's why we were both there. Chris's father-in-law was dying from cancer and had only a short time to live. His wife had taken the kids to Connecticut to spend Christmas with their grandfather and grandmother, but Chris couldn't go because of his standby status.

It was on our third meeting that I asked Chris how and when he knew he was bisexual. He said it all happened just four years before he and I met. He and another engineer, about his age, were sent to Beirut, Lebanon, to make an inspection of a company project. When they arrived at their hotel, even though they had guaranteed reservations, there was no room for them; the hotel had overbooked. While they were talking to the general manager a cancellation came in. However, it was for only one room with just one double bed. The manager checked with three other hotels and it appeared there was nothing available in the city that night, except for this one cancellation. Not having any other choice, the two registered and departed for the same room.

When it came time to retire, sometime after unpacking their bags, they discovered neither had brought pajamas. Each slept in the nude at home and while traveling. It had been a long, hot, sweltering day, and since there was no air conditioning in the hotel, they agreed—to hell with it—they were not going to wear underwear to bed.

In the middle of the night, they awoke and found themselves entwined around each other. Remember, it was only a double bed. The adrenaline began to rise rapidly and so did a couple of other things. Soon, they were fondling each other, and eventually, it reached the point that each had an orgasm. That was the extent of it. According to Chris, there was no oral copulation or anal intercourse, just lots of stroking and fondling. He said that later it seemed there was something lacking that night and he wanted to explore the cause of his erotic feelings about his associate.

Chris said as far as he was concerned, he wasn't born gay and if there was anything in his genes to cause him to become gay, it was strange it didn't manifest itself until his early forties. He didn't know what caused him to react the way he did that night in Beirut. Nevertheless, a short time later he had a compelling urge to have sexual contact with his associate. Chris felt that if that incident in Beirut hadn't happened he may never have been gay as long as he lived.

Prior to that night both he and his associate were as straight as they come. Although the incident in Beirut struck both of them as a little strange and almost bizarre at the time, Chris and his friend developed a bisexual relationship with lots of lustful fire. That experience was his initiation into bisexuality and a turning point in his life. The other fellow was also married and had three children, and they both loved their families dearly.

Chris told me his wife had no conceivable idea of his bisexuality. He was a virile man and was thoroughly convinced that only he satisfied all her sexual needs and desires. All this, in spite of the fact that now he had ongoing sexual relationships with a number of men.

For seven years after meeting Chris in that steam bath on Christmas Day, we would have beautiful, satisfying sexual encounters a couple of times each month. That Christmas Day, in one respect, was a hellish time for my family and me; yet in another respect, it resulted in seven years of marvelous, pleasurable experiences. Eventually, Chris was transferred and he and his family moved to a suburb of Washington, D.C., where he was to work out of an office in the Pentagon.

During the years I was a vice president of the East Bay XYZ Group, I was a member of a national association relating to my field of endeavor. The association sponsored an annual convention in a different city each year, and there was usually a turn out of approximately three hundred members from around the country. The three-day affair was a "field day" for the homos and even the bisexuals, although some of them would have their wives along. It was amazing—if you knew a homo or a bi, he'd introduce you to another, and this would lead to another and another.

One meeting that stands out in my mind was at The Palmer House in downtown Chicago. A good friend of mine, who I will call Dave, and who was also bisexual, was attending the meeting with his wife. We had had many sexual encounters together before, so when the ladies were on a cultural tour of the city, Dave invited me up to his room.

Dave loved to be on the receiving end of anal intercourse, and, when traveling, always carried an enema syringe. I'm sure he had it well hidden from his wife. After we got into his room and got our clothes off, he got the syringe out of a locked briefcase. We went into the bathroom together. Dave took a hotel drinking glass, filled it with warm water, and then filled his syringe. After he did the enema bit, he washed out the syringe in the same glass. Then, we had our fun.

Although Dave was probably a clean and fastidious individual, I think of that hotel-glass incident every time I check into a hotel or motel room. Even though the glasses may have a wrapper or cap on top, I wash out the one I'm going to use with hot sudsy water. I have a phobia for not trusting the sanitary cleanliness of hotel and motel drinking glasses. Most major hotels and some motels run the drinking glasses through a sterilizing machine after each occupancy. However, I don't have confidence in the process because of the caliber of people involved. I even scrub out the ice buckets and have thought of carrying a bottle of isopropyl alcohol to do my own sterilizing routine. I used to think the glass episode, just described, might be a factor in transmitting AIDS. However, my knowledge of the subject in the past two or three years now refutes that idea.

Dave worked in a very large organization similar to mine in San Francisco. Our offices, his in the financial district of the city and mine in downtown Oakland, were separated only by the bay. We didn't let that stop us when we wanted to get together. We were only about thirty to thirty-five minutes apart.

One morning in the fall of 1970, Dave called and asked if we could get together that afternoon at a hotel room that he and two other senior executives in his firm shared the cost of. These three guys split the cost of this room just so they would have a place to take someone when the opportunity presented itself. They had a small locked credenza in the room that served as a bar. In addition to a couple of bottles of booze and mix, Dave kept an old locked attaché case in the cabinet, which contained an enema syringe, a couple of large tubes of K-Y lubricating jelly, and a large water glass used only for filling and cleaning the syringe.

Dave and the other two guys who shared the room were not totally compatible. One was bisexual like Dave and the other straight. He didn't know the other two were bi and they didn't want him to know. The straight guy thought the other two took only ladies to the room. Dave said they had to be very cautious about scheduling use of the room and sometimes it was a little hairy.

As I stated earlier, Dave's favorite sex activity was anal intercourse. When I arrived at the room, he had already used his enema. After showering, Dave told me the straight guy was in an all-day meeting and the bi guy was out of town. Dave had also assured me before that the room was only serviced after it had been used and word was left with the manager. Nonetheless, we were going at it hot and heavy when we heard a key turn in the door. Dave and I froze. To our amazement, it was his bi associate who had arrived back from his trip early and had come by to pick up a cigarette lighter he had left there several days before. He agreed to join us and after taking a shower, we had a three-way party for the next couple of hours, after which, all of us were frazzled.

Once I asked Dave how he managed to pay his share of the room cost without his wife knowing about it. He said it was just a matter of showing three or four guest lunches on his business expense account each month, lunches that didn't take place. He said the head waiters in a couple of restaurants would give him blank customer stubs from luncheon and dinner checks. He would fill them in for the amount needed and turn them in with his expense reports. Dave said, he turned his paycheck over to his wife every two weeks, but the expense check was his.

Not long after joining the XYZ Group, I had to make an overnight trip to Pittsburgh, Pennsylvania. I was at the downtown Gateway Hilton Hotel and about 10:30 P.M. decided to take a little walk for some fresh air. I was about two blocks from the hotel looking in the window of a sporting goods store, when a handsome black guy about my age came by and stopped at the same window. We exchanged a few words, and before long we were engaged in conversation. He had a British accent dripping with the Queen's English. He introduced himself as Cedrick and said he had just gotten off work and was on his way home. It was obvious there was some attraction between us.

It turned out that Cedrick was the maitre d' of a posh downtown restaurant. He was a debonair fellow with light, soft black skin and a contagious smile which went from his chin to his forehead and from ear to ear. Later I learned that he came to this country, seven years before, from the British West Indies. For some reason our vibes seemed to connect that night, and we knew we wanted to get involved with each other. I had always had compelling reservations about taking a stranger to my hotel room, so I told Cedrick I couldn't because my wife was there in bed, although I was really by myself. He said his partner strongly disapproved of bringing home strangers, so we were just about at an impasse. For lack of a better idea, we decided to go to the hotel men's room and appraise each other's "family jewels." We were standing side by side at urinals and it was obvious each of us had something the other wanted; however, our attitude about strangers still prevailed. Finally, Cedrick suggested that we go to a downtown park nearby, which we did. After a brief stroll through the park, we came to a secluded, dimly lit spot and before we knew it, we were having oral sex with each other. We each had orgasms, and Cedrick was all man.

Later, I thought it may have been poor judgment on my part not to have taken Cedrick to my room. However, I have never trusted my evaluation and assessment of character in a situation like that. What I did by going to the park with him was much more perilous than taking him to my room. We were both vulnerable in that situation, but luckily nothing unpleasant happened.

About twenty years ago I had to make a business trip to New York City. I wanted to be in the heart of the action, so I reserved a room at the old Hotel Astor on Times Square, today the site of the fifty-four story One Astor Plaza building at 1515 Broadway. Early on the first evening, I decided to go to Jack Dempsey's Restaurant nearby for dinner. Often Dempsey would sit in a booth at the window and watch the sidewalk crowds stroll by. After dinner I walked back to the Astor. When I got to the hotel, I thought I would go into the bar which was at street level.

After going inside, I was somewhat surprised to find that it was obviously a gay bar. There was only one empty stool at the bar so I sat down there. The guy on my left was absorbed in an intimate conversation with the guy on his left. The guy on my right was day-dreaming, and perhaps just waiting for me. He was a handsome fellow, impeccably dressed, about my size and build, and probably about five years younger. I ordered a scotch and water. Soon we were engrossed in conversation. After about ten minutes, he put his hand on my leg, just above the knee. We talked about five more minutes and then he said he had to go to the restroom. He had placed about $17 in bills on the bar, and he asked me to keep an eye on them until he came back in a few minutes. I later realized this was a ploy to instill his confidence in me and my trust in him. When he returned we resumed our conversation. Soon, we were both ready for another drink and he insisted on buying the round. By this time, his hand was back on my leg and moving higher. The place was alive with frivolity and nobody noticed. By the time we finished our drinks, he had his hand in my crotch and was rubbing my penis. I couldn't take it any longer and invited him up to my room, in spite of my long-standing reservations about welcoming strangers to my hotel room.

I assumed that as soon as we got into the room we would be taking our clothes off. However, immediately after I closed the door, he said, "Let me see your wallet." I replied in astonishment, "You don't want to see my wallet." His face got frightfully flushed and in a loud, commanding tone he said, "Give me your wallet!" I refused again and at that point, he whipped out a switchblade knife from his coat pocket. When I heard the blade click, I thought, oh my God, this is for real. This beautiful man and seemingly nice guy whom I was looking forward to going to bed with had suddenly turned into a thief and a killer. He was not only bent on fleecing me, but also my destruction. The blade on that knife looked like it was two-feet long.

To this day, I believe God told me what to do. After a very rapid thought process, I said, "I don't have much money in my wallet. But in my bag I have $500 in American Express travelers checks. I will endorse them over to you and you can get the cash immediately—you know they're just like cash." I pointed toward my suitcase on a luggage rack. As he turned in that direction, I yanked open the room door and ran down the hall screaming and pounding each door I passed. He panicked, ran into the hall, saw a lighted exit sign at the opposite end, and went in that direction, where he must have run down the fire-escape stairwell.

A guest called the front desk and told them a madman had gone berserk and was creating a disturbance on the ninth floor. Within three or four minutes the house detective or security guard was there. After we discussed the near calamity, he came into my room and called the night manager. He told the manager what had happened and said there could be a reprisal. He said I should be moved to another room on another floor, and that the room I was occupying should remain empty the rest of the night. He stayed with me until a bellman arrived and moved me to another room.

The following morning I checked out of that hotel and into another across town. I had wanted to be in the heart of the action, but never anticipated the danger. It was just a little more action than I really wanted. Since that abominable experience, I have never invited a stranger to my hotel room, nor will I go to the hotel room of a stranger.

Sometimes some of the most intelligent yet naive gays wander into the "jungle." Nine months after my hair-raising experience in a Manhattan hotel, a friend of mine was murdered in his hotel room in Washington, D.C. He was an executive in a San Jose, California, organization similar to mine in Oakland, and we belonged to the same professional association. The day after he was murdered, he was to appear before a congressional transportation committee concerning problems of distribution for California's enormous agricultural industry. I had no gay association with him, but learned from a couple of our mutual friends that he was definitely gay. The murder was never solved, but his closest friends believed that he met a man he was attracted to and invited him to his room. When I think of this, it makes me realize how lucky I was to survive my experience in New York City.

In 1966, at one of the popular gay baths in San Francisco, I met a young man, two or three years younger than myself, whom I'll call Sandy. After we had our sexual fun, we got involved in a lengthy conversation which lasted about an hour and a half. This was the beginning of a long and, pardon the pun, fruitful gay relationship—nine years.

Sandy owned a stylish beauty salon across the bay in Berkeley near the university. For almost nine years, when I was not traveling, I would meet Sandy once a week in his shop after business hours. It was usually after five o'clock and sometimes later. I would call my wife in San Francisco and tell her I was working on a paper project and would be an hour or two late coming home. It wasn't always the same day and I would call her in mid-afternoon to give her a little advance notice. Sandy's shop in Berkeley was only about fifteen minutes from my office in Oakland. He had a little lounge at the rear of the shop, used as a rest area for the operators. In the lounge was a long, soft sofa. Over the years, Sandy and I spent many fun-filled hours on that sofa. It was a funny thing—invariably when I arrived home, Sue would tell me I looked like I had been working too hard; I was exhausted.

Sandy was bisexual, divorced, and had a daughter in her mid teens who lived with her mother. He had a male lover and they were co-owners of a charming little bohemian-style house in the Berkeley hills overlooking San Francisco Bay, the city, and the Golden Gate Bridge. His mate was an intermediate-school teacher and in all those years, I never met Sandy's mate, although I saw him from a distance on a couple of occasions.

Sandy assured me that neither of them were jealous and each had their own extracurricular friendships. I also knew that Sandy had a girlfriend with whom he occasionally had an encounter. Instead of meeting him at his shop, Sandy and I would often meet for lunch, and then we would go to my boat berthed in the Berkeley Marina. I had a thirty-foot sloop (sailboat) complete with head, galley, and sleeping accommodations for six. We would go down into the cabin of the boat, pull the hatch cover closed, and secure the inside lock.

One bright sunny day, Sandy and I were in the cabin of the boat, going at it "hammer and tongs." He had an infatuation for my testicles, and was tonguing my scrotum. They're a little larger than most and "so round and firm and fully packed." Sandy also loved to have me play with his breasts and nipples. Even though he was flat chested, his nipples were large and protruding. They were intensely sensitive and when I would tongue them, it drove him wild. While we were going at it, suddenly we heard someone trying to open the hatch cover. We literally stopped breathing and instantly became as limp as two pieces of wet rope. The effort to open the cover went on for about ten minutes and then we could hear someone climbing out of the cockpit. I looked through an opening in the curtains on one of the ports and saw Sue walking down the float back toward the parking lot. I said to Sandy, "My God, that's my wife! What the hell is she doing here?" Sue didn't see my car in the parking lot because luckily we had come in Sandy's Mercedes. Even though we were two consenting adults, we immediately got dressed, then waited for about fifteen minutes and left.

When I arrived home that evening, Sue said, "The most frustrating thing happened to me today. I drove clear across the bridge to the marina to get my watch I left in a drawer on the boat last Sunday. But when I turned the key in the hatch cover, it jammed and I couldn't get it open." "That's too bad, honey," I replied. Sue went on, "I tried for about ten minutes, but the thing was stuck and I just couldn't turn it. If I had had a key to the locker, I would have tried a little WD-40. Any other time there would be people all over their boats, but I couldn't find anyone to help me." She told me that she had even gone to the harbor master's office, but they were all out to lunch. I promised to go by the boat the next day and bring the watch home that evening. Just another close shave in my life and I've had a few.

While I'm writing about Sandy, I'll tell of a couple of unusual situations. Sometimes the way people get their kicks is a little intriguing. Sandy's mate played the piano. They had a baby grand in front of a large, floor-to-ceiling picture window overlooking the bay. As Sandy told it, his mate loved to play the piano in the nude especially in the evening, by candlelight, with the lights of San Francisco in the distance. He said his mate called it stress therapy. According to Sandy half the time they didn't wear clothes in the house anyway.

One evening in Sandy's shop he wanted to give me a haircut in the nude. So, we both took our clothes off and I did indeed get a haircut in the nude. We played with each other in the process and it was like childish fun. I didn't really think of it as "kinky sex," which I have an aversion toward. I can't stomach the absurdness of the leather and bondage scene or a "drag queen" doing "its" thing in full splendor. And the very thought of sadomasochism makes me ill. That's a weird, bizarre way of getting your sex kicks and only for sick minds. I abhor transsexuals and transvestites. For me, it's very disgusting to see a man in women's clothes, unless he's performing in a show. I know many gay couples have their male and female mate roles, but when one tries so hard to fill the female role, even to the extent of dressing like a woman, that's going way too far. I'm sure the psychiatrists have a pseudoscientific name for it, but to me, it's just kinky sex. I like virile masculine men and tender feminine women.

I remember reading a newspaper account, three or four years ago, and then seeing television coverage of a gay wedding involving two men. I found it grossly disgusting. It seemed like contemptuous mockery of the sacrament of matrimony instituted by Jesus Christ 2000 years ago. I believe that in the next few years, people will become liberal in their views and attitudes toward the gay population. However, I can't quite imagine liberal thinking ever condoning or giving a blessing to gay marriages. Perhaps I'm just a little old fashioned.

In 1972, I flew to Phoenix, Arizona, on business, and during a long wait to check into my hotel, I had to use the men's room off the main lobby. After going in, I opened the door to one of the toilet stalls and closed it behind me. Much to my dismay there was a large "glory hole" in one of the panels separating my toilet from the one on the other side. The hole was perhaps six inches up and down and about four inches wide.

Glory holes are usually found in wood-panel restroom stalls and appear to have been cut through with a small keyhole saw. Most holes have sanded edges. How they got there, no one knows except the guy who did it. The amazing thing is, they often remain for long periods of time. These holes are customarily found in "tearooms," which is gay jargon for public restrooms frequented by gays for fast sex.

A gay man will perform oral copulation through this hole on another man on the other side of the stall. Some guys like the anonymity of this kind of sex, especially closet gays who still consider themselves straight. It seems ridiculously awkward to me, but I have seen even anal intercourse taking place through a glory hole. Glory holes can be found in such places as restrooms in gay bars, steam baths, and major universities. Occasionally, you will see one in a public restroom. I couldn't believe there would be one in the men's room of this Phoenix hotel of such fine repute.

The gay who solicits fellatio through a glory hole is taking a real risk, in more ways than one. First of all, he has no probable idea as to whether or not the guy he is soliciting is safe, from a health standpoint. Secondly, in such an environment and setting there is the constant fear of intrusion and police arrest, unless you have "scouts." And then, there is the possibility that the guy on the other side is a macho straight and will crush your hands or break your nose. However, most gays who engage in this type of thing have a sixth sense for good or bad vibes from the guy on the other side and act accordingly.

While sitting on the "John," a motioning hand came through the hole. Sure enough, someone was on the other side and wanted to make contact. Now, I was getting hot and horny. When I finished my chore, I glanced through the hole and saw a pleasant-looking young man. His hand came through the hole again. At this point I was developing a stiff erection, and despite the risks, I eased toward the hole in the wall. Instantly he had my penis in his mouth. After three or four minutes of reverberating action, I had a climax in his mouth. Then, I dried myself with toilet paper, pulled up my pants, went to a wash basin, washed my hands, and was on my way, much relieved of many tensions. I undoubtedly left someone behind who had also been satisfied. Later in the day, I wondered how many mouthfuls that guy may have taken that morning. That evening I learned that the hotel's cocktail lounge was a quasi-gay bar and the men's room was a hub of homo activity.

For a number of years I had been involved in considerable domestic travel and often was gone from home for ten days to two weeks at a time. In 1972, for my birthday, my wife gave me a membership in Playboy Clubs International. She went all out and gave me a gold (charge) card, knowing that Playboy Clubs were strictly a man's domain and that I wouldn't be exposed to "bar flies" on the make. And, of course, she never suspected my interest in men, but at that time, my bisexuality hadn't progressed to the point that I might try to pick up a guy in a straight bar. I'm sure Sue didn't think the bunnies in the clubs would be a threat to my fidelity and she was so right. Eventually I was in eleven of the twenty-two hutches in the bunny club empire. It didn't seem to make any difference where they were— Chicago, New York, San Francisco, or Los Angeles—the bunnies, at least a major portion of them, had eyes only for one another. It was so obvious that many of those girls were lesbian. For the most part, they were beautiful creatures abounding in feminine pulchritude, yet they had an impassive, impervious personality, except when you might observe them consorting among themselves.

Of the many times I was in Playboy Clubs across the country, there were perhaps only three or four occasions when I felt my bar or table waitress exhibited any attention to me or my guests as males. There were a number of times when my guests observed the situation just as I did and even commented about it. Many of those girls, as pretty as they were, were insensitive to the male patrons. It seemed that even the straight girls were caught up in acknowledging the glances and mutual admiration of the others.

One time while having dinner by myself in one of the clubs, even though I realized it could cause a confrontation, I asked my bunny, "Are you a lesbian?" Her reply was, "What do you think?" I felt I had obviously gotten my answer. I told her I was gay and it was only a matter of inquisitiveness on my part. From then on, she exuded cordiality and I got undivided attention. At one point, she brought one of her cohorts over to my table and introduced her to me. I felt like a VIP celebrity. Most gays and lesbians hang together because of our inglorious genesis.

Someone once said that all lesbians have mannish mannerisms and characteristics. That's pure nonsense and the homo-sexual Playboy bunnies attested to that. Some of the most gorgeous, beautiful women I have known were admitted lesbians.

4

Science Peers into the Closet and Gay Liberation Begins

Nearly fifty years ago an extensive and far-reaching research project on human sexual behavior was undertaken by the eminent scientist Alfred C. Kinsey, a professor of zoology at Indiana University. In this broad and exhaustive undertaking, Kinsey was assisted by renowned men and women in various fields of endeavor, including psychiatrists, psychologists, sociologists, biologists, physicians, and various clinicians. More than 12,000 people contributed data for this vast research project. For the last six years of the project, Kinsey was supported by the National Research Council's Committee for Research on Problems of Sex, with funds granted by the Medical Sciences Division of the Rockefeller Foundation in New York City.

In 1948, the first of the acclaimed Kinsey reports was published. It was titled *Sexual Behavior in the Human Male*. A subsequent report was titled *Sexual Behavior in the Human Female*. In his preface to the first publication, Dr. Alan Gregg of the Rockefeller Foundation eloquently expressed his opinion that the world was in dire need of scientific knowledge about the subject of sex.

The Kinsey reports were published as textbooks and reference material, and were primarily intended for medical doctors, psychiatrists, sociologists, marriage counselors, and other professionals. However, if there had been a "best seller" designation in those days, Dr. Kinsey's books would probably have ridden the crest for at least a couple of years. The popularity of the reports was a powerful indication that the American people felt a compelling need for knowledge about human sexuality. In reality, the Kinsey reports are boring reading for the average layman, unless one has a penchant for analyzing charts and graphs and assimilating technical data. The present book conveys a more intimate insight into the activities and lifestyle of the gay world than either of the Kinsey books. I am writing in a vernacular that should give most readers a comprehensive understanding of homosexuality and gay life. The word "gay" was just coming into being when the first Kinsey report was published. The researchers possibly felt the terminology wouldn't stick and it isn't to be found anywhere in the voluminous reports. Likewise, the word "queer" is not found in the reports. This is understandable since the findings were the culmination of a technical, scientific research project and the only nomenclature for homosexual was homosexual.

Only a small portion of the overall nine-year Kinsey research project was devoted to the homosexual. At the time the Kinsey researchers were compiling their data, a large segment of society considered homosexuals to be mentally deranged and harboring criminal intentions. As a matter of fact, homosexual acts were then legally regarded as criminal offenses, regardless of consenting adults. The Kinsey reports indicate that many of the homosexual histories were inconclusive. It was difficult in those days (and remember, this is not so long ago) to get homosexuals to talk candidly about their feelings, desires, sexual activities, or their lifestyle as a whole. They lived in constant fear of harassment by the law and the consequential wrath of the courts. To be a homosexual then was to live a frightening, haunting existence.

In the ensuing years, the United States Supreme Court has taken a more lenient stance regarding the medieval, archaic sex laws that once restrained our God-given human rights. Most states and local jurisdictions have followed suit. Now consenting adults may do whatever they wish, sexually, in the privacy of their own bedroom. It really wasn't that big a thing to me. I never had visions of my wife being hauled away by police, in handcuffs, because she was caught "going down" on me. However, in a more serious vein, the loosening of legal restraints has relieved untold mental anguish and frustration among gays.

The Kinsey findings on human sexual behavior caused a worldwide hoopla. I remember it vividly, even though it took place more than forty years ago. The Kinsey researchers were baffled in their attempt to understand the biological and social origins of homosexuality, and they often referred to it as a rare phenomenon. Hormonal and hereditary factors, as well as neurotic and psychopathic behavior, were ruled out as causes of homosexuality. I believe this excerpt from the first Kinsey report has extraordinary significance:

> In these terms (of physical contact to the point of orgasm), the data in the present study indicate that at least 37 percent of the male population has some homosexual experience between the beginning of adolescence and old age. This is more than one male in three of the persons one may meet as he passes along a city street.*

The Kinsey reports shed some long overdue light on the matter of homosexuality. Nevertheless, I believe the Kinsey

---

*Excerpt reprinted with permission of the Kinsey Institute, Indiana University.

researchers saw only the tip of the iceberg in regard to the homosexual, and Dr. Kinsey, who died in 1956, probably never realized what a meaningful contribution his research made to the homosexual cause. I suppose you might say Dr. Kinsey was a man ahead of his time.

At about the same time the first Kinsey report was published, the gay underground was becoming restless. Gays were observing the bold clashes of black civil rights activists who were lashing out at white society after generations of degrading and painful oppression. The prejudice that blacks endured was similar to what gays experienced. Openly admitted homosexuals, for the most part, could not get employment and jobs that matched their educational qualifications, talents, and abilities. They were stereotyped into such occupations as hairdresser, interior decorator, floral arranger, fashion designer, male secretary, waiter, and hospital orderly. This was very much like the stereotyping that "Negroes" experienced when they were confined to occupations such as janitor, domestic porter, bootblack, and prizefighter.

Gay culture was emerging and was becoming a cohesive factor among gays who were being attracted to certain geographic communities, usually in the larger metropolitan cities. New York's Christopher Street and San Francisco's Castro Street were and still are good examples of these cohesive gay hubs. These districts were not exactly the "Beverly Hills" of the metropolitan centers, and sometimes were dismissively referred to as gay ghettos. However, you must bear in mind that there are thousands upon thousands of "closet" gays who never set foot in those urban centers, men and women who live in other areas of the cities and suburban environs.

In the late 1940s and early 1950s, gay bars were becoming popular and beginning to appear just about everywhere. Like any other social entity, gay people congregate in order to meet one another. Straight people had long had the singles bars and now it was time for the gay bar scene to develop, where gays could meet, make acquaintances, and develop friendships. Gay bars caught on very rapidly since there was no acceptable place for gays to socialize at that time, other than the baths. It is estimated there are between four to five thousand gay bars in the United States today. You can always be sure to find them near any large military base or major university.

Not long after World War II, there seemed to be a rudimentary awakening of homosexuals. Those individuals who were then called queer, because of their sexual preference, were becoming indignant about their disreputable distinction. They knew they were not mentally ill, depraved perverts, or a danger to society. However, the long arm of the law treated them that way, and they were often harassed, intimidated, terrorized, and physically assaulted by law enforcement officers. For generations, homosexuals had hidden in the "closet." But now the "closet" was seething with bitterness, resentment, and even outrage.

Dr. Kinsey's published research reports were reassuring to homosexuals. Each one knew he was not alone; there were hundreds of thousands and even millions like him. Gays began to organize and form coherent survival groups. Some of the organizations that were formed, some even before the formal start of the gay liberation movement, were: Gay Activists Alliance (GAA), New York's Gay Liberation Front, Mattachine Society and Foundation, Homophile Effort for Legal Protection (HELP), Knights of the Clock, San Francisco's Society for Individual Rights (SIR), Daughters of Bilitis (lesbian), Society for Mutual Equality (SAME), ONE, Inc., Columbia University's Student Homophile League, the Mandrake Society, and the North American Conference of Homophile Organizations (NACHO), just to name a few. NACHO attempted to be the pivotal core of all homophile (homosexual) organizations. By the mid 1960s, there were dozens upon dozens of these groups across the country. The time was fast approaching for a well defined gay liberation movement.

In 1968, the Reverend Troy Perry, a compassionate but bold

Pentecostal preacher, realized the compelling need for an unbiased, interdenominational gay religious organization. Perry had been married, was the father of two sons, and had served as pastor of congregations in Florida and California before renouncing his pastoral and marital responsibilities in 1963. He explained his separation from family and ministry as a recognition of his homosexuality. Perry is a powerful, persuasive, articulate speaker. He founded the Metropolitan Community Church, a strictly gay religious organization. It all started with a handful of worshipers in a private home in Los Angeles. Today the Metropolitan Community Church (MCC) has branches in just about every major city in the United States. You will find it listed in the white pages of the telephone book. It's a place where scrupulous, virtuous gays, as well as those who want to avoid the bar scene, can congregate and fraternize and at the same time add some spiritual strength to their lives. Troy Perry has made one of the greatest contributions to the homosexual cause. He is known as the "Martin Luther Queen" of the gay culture.

As the gay liberation movement was progressing underground, the leaders and activists were learning strategy from the black organizations, principally the National Association for the Advancement of Colored People (NAACP). There was almost an alliance between black groups and gay groups, both of which were attempting to overcome their social and legal oppression. Gays have an advantage in one respect. On the surface, it's usually not clear whether a person is gay or straight. However, there's no disguising race. Nevertheless, the black culture has had the greatest impact upon the initiation of social change of any of the minorities in the United States in the twentieth century.

By early 1969, gays around the country had become infuriated with the decades of police harassment and entrapment. The brutal invasion of privacy in the form of attacks by vice squads and their humiliating consequences had become insufferable. The boiling point was reached on June 28, 1969, when a police raid on the Stonewall Inn, a gay bar in New York's Greenwich Village, erupted into a rampaging riot. The organized gay underground exploded into the open, determined no longer to be intimidated, hassled, and then mollified. A two-day street battle ensued, with police at times barricading themselves against the onslaught of the resisting gay "troops." Simple resistance to a police raid turned into an all-out combat offensive for a human-rights cause, resulting in costly property damage and bodily injury. Articles about the Stonewall riot appeared in the *New York Times* on June 29, June 30, and again on July 3, 1969. This wild insurrection, referred to as the "Stonewall Rebellion," is looked upon today as the decisive start and birthday of the gay liberation movement in this country.

The October 31, 1969, issue of *Time* magazine gave its front cover to an article titled "The Homosexual in America." The article was almost sympathetic with the plight of the homosexual. It was the first of many articles and stories in national publications giving recognition to the homosexual cause. Prior to that, the media shunned the very word homosexual. In the past twenty years, there have been innumerable gay rallies, protests, demonstrations, parades, and conventions around the country. Now gays have become a motivating, decisive factor in many political elections and their support is sought for various other causes. Unfortunately, many of the older gay activists have become complacent and feel that the "fire" has gone out of the fight. I hope there are enough that realize the battle isn't over yet.

The Stonewall Rebellion gave encouragement to gays in other parts of the country to resist harassment. For instance, in San Francisco many of the street gays who congregated in Union Square, in the heart of the city, used to gravitate to the men's room on the basement level of Macy's department store across the street. The spot soon became a "tea room." Eventually the situation became a burdensome aggravation to Macy's security people, and in the summer of 1970, after long surveillance, Macy's own plainclothes detectives arrested forty men for their homosexual activities in that restroom. San Francisco's Society for Individual Rights (SIR), a daringly activist and innovative organization, took on Macy's. SIR organized a picketing demonstration on the sidewalks of the store to protest the arrest of the forty gays. Soon SIR intensified its pressure by organizing a national boycott of the chain, but the effort really never gained steam and in a short time fizzled out.

Since the Stonewall Rebellion, gay bars have been a focal point in the liberation movement. They are not what they used to be—a clandestine rendezvous where a few of the more outward and brazen gay people sought out one another in secret. In 1974, perhaps the most notable and prestigious gay night club and disco opened in West Hollywood at the edge of Beverly Hills. Its name—Studio One. Because of its size, popularity, and patronage by celebrities, it has done much to make the gay lifestyle an acceptable part of American culture. It's an awesome place, featuring four separate cocktail lounges, a video theater, and a discotheque the size of a basketball court. As many of 1,200 to 1,400 people pass through this colossal "watering hole" on a Saturday night. Studio One boasts of having had as its guests at one time or another such luminaries as Nancy Reagan and her intimate friend Betsy Bloomingdale, Burt Reynolds, Liza Minnelli, Richard Chamberlain, Barbra Streisand, Candice Bergen, Johnny Mathis, Elizabeth Taylor, Fred Astaire, Ginger Rogers, Carol Channing, Steve Allen, Carol Burnett, Gene Kelly, Johnny Carson, and many, many more. Raquel Welch was once seen dancing with her boyfriend among the crowds of men dancing with men and women dancing with women. In March 1984, Joan Rivers did a fund-raising benefit show for AIDS research to a standing-room-only, sellout audience at Studio One. Today, to encounter celebrities in a gay bar or club is nothing new. They may be there only to satisfy their curiosity, but the fact that they are unconcerned about being seen in a gay bar is a testament to their acknowledgment of gay status and their acceptance of gay establishments.

By the late 1970s and early '80s, the gay liberation movement had made its impact. San Francisco now, unquestionably, had the dubious distinction of being the gay capital of the country. It is estimated that between 1974 and 1978 more than 20,000 gay men had migrated to the city. By 1980, two out of five adult males in San Francisco were openly gay. The city was a constant hub of gay activities, including parades, marches, and demonstrations that would attract hundreds of thousands of people. These gatherings always brought out the exhibitionists. On hand for most events was a group of drag queens who dressed as nuns and called themselves the "Sisters of Perpetual Indulgence." Los Angeles was also fast becoming a mecca of gay activities. In June 1980, California's Governor Edmund G. (Jerry) Brown, Jr.—a perennial bachelor—issued a proclamation honoring Gay Freedom Week throughout the state. Brown is now making another serious run for the White House, and there is still no prospective First Lady at his side.

Today, nearly two decades after the start of the formal gay liberation movement, the gay world is well organized and efficiently coordinated. The index to the 1987 (twenty-first edition) of the *Encyclopedia of Associations* lists among more than 23,000 national and international organizations 134 gay and lesbian groups in the United States. A small cross section of the organizations is as follows: Gay Academic Union, Gay Press Association, Association of Gay and Lesbian Psychiatrists, Federal Lesbians and Gays, Lesbian and Gay Caucus of the Democratic National Committee, Gay Mormons United, Children of Gay Parentage, National Coalition of Black Lesbians and Gays, Gay People in Medicine, Gay American Indians, Presbyterian Gay Caucus, Spouses of Gays Association (straight), Gay People in Christian Science, Gay Veterans Association, Federation of Parents and Friends of Lesbians and Gays, World Congregation of Gay and Lesbian Jewish Organizations, Gay Nurses' Alliance, Gay Episcopalians and Their Friends, Association of Lesbian and Gay Psychologists, Gay Fathers Coalition, United Church of Christ Gay Caucus, Gay Actors' Alliance, and Institution for the Protection of Lesbian and Gay Youth. Most of the organizations have branches or chapters in many of the major cities around the country. Obviously, in the more recent years of gay liberation, lesbians have also become more vociferous.

5

Family Life as Husband and Father

In the past ten years or so, I have lost my deep-seated guilt complex regarding bisexuality. Even though I don't feel comfortable enough to reveal this facet of my personality, life has been much easier with far less trepidation in recent years. There have been times in the past, however, when the anxiety, torment, stress, and frustration were unbearable. I suppose all this has made a better man of me. I know I'm much more compassionate now than I was twenty or thirty years ago. Then I sometimes felt like a caged stud bull that wanted to take on the whole world; yet every Sunday morning I was in church with my wife, son, and daughter.

Regardless of our incompatibility from a sexual standpoint, my wife has always been my champion and my greatest inspiration and motivator through the years. Sue was always up when the chips were down, except for that miserable Christmas Eve many years ago. She truly does love me; we're just not on the same sexual wavelength. She can take it or leave it and most of the time would just as soon leave it. She is not exuberant about sex. I love to go down (cunnilingus) on her, but she shows no reaction. And certainly there's no reciprocation. I've done it to other women and it drives them to a state of frenzied ecstasy—not so with my wife. Sue grew up in a stricter, more puritanical environment than I did, and perhaps this has a bearing on her sexual attitude, even now.

There is something strange about the whole thing, however. Sue and I were high school sweethearts. The year before we were married, while I was in the navy, we slept together many times in hotels and motels in San Diego, Los Angeles, and San Francisco. She would die if our kids ever found out. She was a sexy girl then, but it all changed after the birth of our first child. And when number two arrived, our son Mark, I became number four in terms of priority. She was a young wife and mother, trying to keep a household going on a limited budget. I suppose as her domestic responsibilities grew and the workday got longer, her desire for sexual pleasure diminished. Within five years she wasn't the sexually alive girl I had married. There were times in the early years of our marriage when I seriously thought of divorce. However, it didn't take long for me to get that out of my head, because I couldn't bear the thought of another man raising my son and daughter. I came to the conclusion that there is something more precious in this world than sex. Nevertheless, I found the sex elsewhere.

During the years we were raising our family, our home was a wholesome, innocent environment. The dress code for the kids at home was almost as proper as it was at their parochial schools. Sue was outwardly a prudish girl, who would not tolerate foul language or improper conduct. Our kids weren't even allowed to say "shut up" to their little playmates. This provoked the wrath of mother. Anything more repulsive and deplorable would call for a serious reprimand. Sue's contention is that cursing and the use of improper or profane language is a sign of unstable character and lack of vocabulary. And I do acquiesce in her virtuous thinking.

After we had been married about twelve years, Sue had

to have a hysterectomy. I was happy and even excited about it because I thought it would change our sex lives, knowing that she wouldn't have to worry about pregnancy any longer. In the ensuing years, the hysterectomy had no bearing whatsoever on her sexual desires. I had hopes that when our daughter left home and then our son, our sex lives would return to normal, hopefully like the days before marriage. But that hasn't happened.

Shortly before Sue and I were married, a couple of her girl-friends gave her a bridal shower. There were about twenty-five or thirty women there, young and old. At one point, everyone was given a 3×5 card and asked to write something they would like to have Sue remember. A few months later she showed me the cards. The various suggestions covered everything from helpful advice to gourmet recipes. One old family friend wrote on her card, "Keep your man happy in the bedroom. If he gets all he needs and wants at home, he won't be looking for it elsewhere." I somehow feel there is truth and understanding in that sage advice.

About twenty years ago, Sue and I were at a lavish social function, where there happened to be a professional psychic palm reader. She took my hand and, after scrutinizing the lines in the palm for a few seconds, said, "You are a very passionate man." Obviously, she knew something my wife has never found out or perhaps refuses to recognize. Many women never k ow their husbands, even after thirty and forty years. Beside the sexual imbalance, Sue and I lead a normal life together as man and wife.

When our son was eleven years old, he joined the Boy Scouts. It was obvious from the beginning that Mark would run the full gamut. Even at that tender age he displayed a tenacious sense of responsibility and determination. As predicted, he went through the ranks and after five years was awarded his Eagle. Mark was in a very active and industrious San Francisco troop. His young, vigorous, and energetic Scoutmaster had been an

Eagle Scout just ten years before and now was an intermediate school teacher.

Mark's summer camp, where he spent a week for five consecutive years, was located ninety miles north of San Francisco in a forested area near the beautiful Russian River, a short distance from where it flows into the Pacific Ocean. Nearby is the world-renowned Bohemian Grove, the summer retreat of San Francisco's eminent Bohemian Club, where professional men, corporate czars, political giants, statesmen, and world leaders gather for informal conferences. It's situated in a magnificent two hundred-acre grove of towering coastal redwood trees.

I often felt I became as much absorbed in scouting as my son. For two summers I spent a full week at Mark's scout camp as acting Assistant Scoutmaster. They were character-forming years for Mark and years that created father-son experiences and memories that I shall always cherish. When Mark was awarded his Eagle in a touching, nostalgic ceremony, I felt I had also earned mine. Since I didn't have a father in my formative years, I believe I went overboard to be a good dad to my son. Even though Mark is a young man of the world now, he will always be my little boy. I think most men who are good fathers to their sons feel that way.

Although Mark grew up and was raised in a cosmopolitan metropolis, he was exposed to many provincial advantages. He was involved in exhilarating sports and cultural programs. We spent countless hours fishing and sailing on San Francisco Bay in our elegant thirty-foot sloop. Mark would usually have a girlfriend and/or some of his buddies along. Of course, dad was always there to oversee the safety of the boat and its occupants. Many times mom was there, too. She referred to herself as the "galley slave" and there was always lots of satisfying, good food. In the ski seasons we spent many long fabulous weekends on the slopes of Lake Tahoe and family holiday vacations at California's Mammoth Mountain. There was also scouting with its numerous weekend outings and camping excursions. I'm sure Mark had a more fulfilling youth than a boy who grew up in a suburban or rural atmosphere with a father who had no interest.

When the kids were growing up, we were a close family and all looked out for one another. When Mark was twelve and thirteen, he had a *San Francisco Chronicle/Examiner* newspaper route. If he and I were on a scouting weekend together, his sister and/or mom would deliver his papers and this was no easy chore, since the Sunday paper was usually a handful. There were many fun times with both my son and daughter that bring to mind treasured recollections. Still, dad wasn't exactly a soft touch and there was a no-nonsense respect for discipline in our home. At the same time, if the kids were faced with a predicament or crisis, I was always there to help and with an understanding attitude.

When Margie was away at boarding school, dad was there on father-daughter weekends. When Mark attended an out-of-state university, his mom and I visited him early in his first semester. While having lunch with him in the cafeteria, a number of young men and women stopped at our table to introduce themselves as his friends. It was obvious Mark was already popular on campus.

It's sad that people who become involved in such activities as scouting, boys' clubs, Big Brothers, and Big Sisters are suspected, by some, of being there only to sexually exploit their charges. Granted, you'll read of such criminal acts in the newspapers now and then, but it isn't the norm. In the five years I was involved in scouting, I never saw anything that would arouse suspicion of child molestation on the part of the adults involved and this included the scouting professionals at summer camp. If such an activity had been discovered or detected, regardless of my gay orientation, I would have been just as outraged as any other parent.

When I was growing up, there was some amount of love and affection in my home; however, I feel that since I didn't have a father my mother went overboard not to smother me with her love and affection. There is such a thing as "smother love" and I have seen situations that cause me to believe young men who are exposed to it turn out to be effeminate. You've heard it said, he was a "mama's boy" and sometimes "mama's boys" remain boyish and don't mature into masculine, virile men.

At any rate, and possibly as a result of this, I went too far in controlling and inhibiting my outward love and affection for my son. I never gave him a bear hug or a kiss on the lips after he was four or five years old. Really sad, isn't it? I didn't want him to be a "sissy" or a "queer." I suspected I was gay, and at that point in life I wasn't sure it was such a good thing. Whether gay or straight, why do men have to be so macho? I realize now what an unforgivable mistake it has been and how it has deprived Mark and me for many, many years from openly expressing our love and affection for each other.

My daughter, Margie, is a beautiful young woman, but then I'm prejudiced. She very much resembles her mother when Sue was that age. Margie also had a fulfilling childhood, just as her brother did. Her mother constantly had her involved in various types of projects and programs. In her mid teens, she spent two years in an exclusive girls' boarding school. Margie is a very talented young lady, dedicated mother, and even a gourmet cook. She and her husband, Don, have blessed Sue and me with five beautiful grandchildren, three sons and two daughters; the oldest is seventeen and the youngest eight. I have had some great experiences with my grandkids. We have been camping, fishing, water skiing, and snow skiing. I have been a merit-badge counselor for the two boys involved in scouting and have been on hand for numerous soccer, baseball, and basketball practices and games.

Margie met Don in college and two years later, when she

was twenty-one, they were married. Sue and I gave them a resplendent nuptial mass wedding, followed by an opulent reception for ninety guests at the old prestigious St. Francis Yacht Club in San Francisco. Don is as handsome as Margie is pretty. He comes from a fine middle-income San Francisco family (four sons and two daughters). Today, Don is a young self-made California millionaire. He did it all by himself in thirteen years—well, maybe with a little help from God and Margie at his side. He is president of his own prosperous company which employs more than thirty people, and an incessant worker, shrewd investor, and a bountiful provider for his family.

Don and Margie are globe-trotters, but despite all their travels, they are never gone more than two weeks at a time, and the kids are well taken care of in their absence by the live-in housekeeper. Margie needs the respite she gets when she and Don are traveling or on their mini-vacations three or four times a year. She lives for her kids and husband and is on the go from early morning till late at night. Margie has her kids involved in a myriad of activities and she goes at an unrelenting pace to meet all of their demanding schedules. She is too domesticated to be the socialite type.

Margie's brother is a decided success in his own right. Early in college he plotted his future and today is doing exactly what he set out to do and loves doing so much. Mark got his degree in a field of endeavor that prepared him well for his chosen career and the administrative position he now holds. In his mid thirties, Mark is still not married, and may never be, though he's a handsome guy. He says he may be too set in his ways now to start sharing life with someone else. According to popular mythology, all handsome, unmarried men are gay. Of course, that's a "crock of bull," yet I have wondered many times whether or not my son is gay. If so, he's bisexual, not homosexual. Mark has had many girlfriends in recent years. Three years ago, his mother and I were certain he was ready to take the leap and get married. Then, suddenly after many months, the romance cooled. Mark's sister has made up for his deficiency in providing us with grandchildren.

As the patriarch of this traditional, three-generation family, I am understandably nervous about my secret gay life. The consequences of discovery can be devastating. A friend of mine came to this rude awakening several years ago. He was the exemplification of the All-American family man, yet he was bisexual. He and his wife had been married nineteen years and had a seventeen-year-old son and fifteen-year-old daughter, when his secret was exposed. He had a profound love for his family in spite of his secret gay activities, and was totally involved in raising his kids, including church, academic, social, and sports activities. When his wife discovered conclusive evidence of his bisexuality, the woman became an atrocious ogre and soon wanted a divorce. Even after nineteen years of togetherness and two beautiful kids, there was no reasoning, compassion, or understanding in any member of his family. The revelation of his bisexuality was a humiliation and mortification. His son and daughter, because of the narrow-minded religious and social mores he had helped to instill in them, rejected their father and are now alienated from him. Today he is a broken man; he can't cope with the loss of his family.

The knowledge of this sad experience has haunted me since the day I learned of it. Regardless of my bisexuality I have and will continue to work hard at being a good husband and worthy father. It's a scary thought that the disclosure of my two-sided sexual personality could result in the loss of my family. Even though this is a threatening possibility, I could never be prepared for it. I would like to believe that if my wife and family came to know how my sexuality evolved and the consequences of certain events on my psyche, I would be vindicated.

Nonetheless, if my sexual orientation and escapades were found out by my son, daughter, and grandkids, they would be more troubled and perplexed than the millions of Little Leaguers and fans of Pete Rose when they learned the truth about him—after all, he was their hero. But he did commit a breach of moral standards. No doubt about it—if my secret bisexual life was found out, it would be perceived as moral turpitude and a shameless violation of decency and virtue.

When Margie was a high school senior and Mark was an eighth-grader, I took Sue and them with me on a two-week business trip to the east. We had planned for it several weeks in advance. For me it was a combination of business and vacation. A month prior to the trip I was able to get tickets from our congressman for a guided congressional tour of the White House in Washington. While in the Capitol, we attended a session of Congress from the House Gallery. We saw most of the significant monuments and made a trek to the top of the Washington Monument where we got a bird's-eye view of the city. In the National Archives we saw the Declaration of Independence and the Constitution. The noble, honorable atmosphere and character of the Supreme Court had an impact on all of us. At Arlington National Cemetery we saw the changing of the guard at the Tomb of the Unknown Soldier and the eternal flame on the grave of President John F. Kennedy. For Margie and her mom we made a tour of the Smithsonian Institute. For Mark we saw a shooting exhibition at the firing range in the basement of the FBI headquarters building. Our enriching, cultural tour included a day and a half I had to spend in Philadelphia where probing, adventuresome Mark stuck a finger in the crack of the Liberty Bell in Independence Hall.

In my job at XYZ I had made friends with the west coast trade representative of the New York Port Authority. His office was in San Francisco. At that time the port maintained two helicopters for taking dignitaries and certain visitors on tours of port facilities. Two weeks before we left on our eastern trip my friend made arrangements for my family and me to be taken on a lofty tour of Manhattan Island. We boarded the choppers at the heliport on top of the port's midtown headquarters building. Sue and Margie were in one and Mark and I in the other. From the air we saw the site, at the edge of the Hudson River, where excavation and pile driving had started prior to construction of the port's 110-story, twin-tower World Trade Center, today a major attraction in the Big Apple. Our pilots hovered in the face of the Statue of Liberty, and we got a close-up look at the grand old lady. We went to the observation level atop the 102-story Empire State Building and, on Wall Street, to the New York Stock Exchange during trading hours. We saw a Broadway play, "Hello Dolly," and the dynamic Rockettes at the awesome Radio City Music Hall. We strolled past Carnegie Hall on our way to take a carriage ride through Central Park. We attended Sunday Mass at St. Patrick's Cathedral. Sue had an opportunity to browse through Bloomingdale's and Saks Fifth Avenue.

In Boston, we saw most of the historic sites and monuments. We saw the Boston Pops in concert at Symphony Hall with maestro Arthur Fiedler conducting, and in nearby Cambridge, we took a drive through the campus of Harvard University. Our entire trip was by first-class air with thirteen pieces of luggage. Mark was the major-domo of dunnage. It was a memorable experience, one I'm sure none of us will ever forget. I have tried so hard to be a good husband and benevolent dad in spite of my heterogeneous character and temperamental disposition.

The summer our son was a Life Scout, his mother and I reworked our budget so we could send him on a one-month tour of Europe, which included the Scandinavian countries, England, West Germany, Italy, and France. It was dubbed the Bridge of Friendship Tour and involved forty-three senior scouts from the San Francisco Bay Area Council. In a number of countries and cities visited, the boys were guests in the homes of families of foreign scouts. It was a reciprocation from European scouts who had toured this country two years before and were guests in the homes of American scouts. Mark returned with many photos and souvenirs, and he described the tour as an unforgettable educational and cultural adventure. Sue and I were so glad we could make it possible.

When I did extensive domestic travel for the XYZ Group, I never made a trip I didn't bring home gifts for Sue and the kids. Sometimes I'd spend hours in the evenings or on a weekend shopping for just the right thing for each of them. Sue's gift may have been a dress or blouse or piece of costume jewelry from Neiman-Marcus in Dallas, Saks Fifth Avenue in New York, or Marshall Field in Chicago. I didn't do it because I had a guilt complex about my secret double life. I'm sure I would have done the same thing if I were arrow straight. I love my family—always have and always will.

For my kids and everyone else I worked diligently to portray the role model of a decent, respectable father and husband. At the same time, my impressionable son and daughter were witnessing the total disregard for decency and law and order in this country. In San Francisco in the mid '60s we lived within ten minutes of the infamous Haight/Ashbury district, the commune megalopolis of the country's hippie culture. The district had a constant plume of marijuana smoke drifting overhead in the streets. Pot and psychedelic drugs were available everywhere. The sexual revolution was in full swing. Across the bay in Berkeley, the University of California campus was a war zone with frequent clashes between Vietnam War protesters and the California National Guard. At times National Guard helicopters would strafe protester demonstrations on campus with debilitating gas. We lived within sight of Guard helicopters patrolling the campus of San Francisco State University, where President S. I. Hayakawa was forced a number of times to barricade himself in his office to evade rock-throwing demonstrators. As you may recall, Dr. Hayakawa was later rewarded, by the voters, with a stint in congress as a California senator.

In San Francisco you're close to everything; you can drive from one end of the city to the other in twenty or so minutes. We also lived a short distance from the Castro district—the haven of homosexuality, where gays openly and disgustingly flaunted their way of life. Gay liberation had become a bold reality. The entire country was seething in upheaval; it was almost a revolution against respect for law, order, and morality by hundreds of thousands of young people coast to coast. For Sue and me these were difficult and trying times living so close to the action and at the same time endeavoring to instill honor and integrity in a vulnerable son and daughter. Nevertheless, our efforts paid off.

Early in chapter 1, I briefly referred to a life-long friend who has been like a brother to me. I first knew him in grammar school. Our wives became friends in high school. He doesn't have the slightest idea of my gay orientation. His two daughters and my son and daughter have been very close through the years. Today, our grandkids consider themselves make-believe cousins. We've had some wonderful family times together.

In the early 1980s my friend and I chartered a forty-foot sloop for a seven-day foursome sailing excursion with our wives in the Caribbean, just prior to the hurricane season. Two days out of our home port on St. Vincent Island, an early, unexpected, fierce hurricane hit—Hurricane Allan. For fourteen scary hours we endured a harrowing experience and most of it at night. I really felt that God was our skipper; there was no damage to the boat or physical injuries. We were sailing together with another foursome, two couples, on a similar boat. One of those ladies, the wife of my wife's cousin, could not swim and came close to losing her life. She lost her grip and fell while climbing a rope ladder in an attempt to board a freighter. She finally made it. Two days later when we saw the devastation Allan left on an island we visited, we all realized how lucky we were to be alive. There was some solemn praying on our boat that night and I'm sure God heard it. There were only minor psychological hurts and it was obvious God had been looking after all eight of us. All our kids had been watching Allan's havoc and destruction on TV and reading about it in the papers. They were thoroughly distraught and had visions of us going to the bottom—Davy Jones' Locker. It was two days before we could get to a telephone. Our son and daughter were much relieved to hear our voices.

Sometime ago my wife and I attended our fortieth high school reunion in the town where we were both born and raised. Ours was a large school with an enrollment of over 3,000. There were more than 700 students in our class and about 200 attended the reunion, either single, with their spouse, or a guest. You will recall, I left high school between my junior and senior year to join the navy in World War II. So, in reality, it was Sue's fortieth class reunion.

The nostalgic affair was held in our hometown's most popular hostelry. At one point my champagne consumption was building up pressure and I decided to relieve myself of some of the excess. As I entered the men's room, I was aware that someone was close behind, almost on my heels. There were four urinals on the wall. I stepped up to one and the guy behind strode up to the one beside me. We exchanged some cordial remarks and then the vibes emerged. I glanced over and he had a fixed stare on my "you know what." I looked down at "his" and then we made eye contact. We stood there for an inordinate amount of time, perhaps three or four minutes—much longer than it would have taken either of us to empty our bladder. We backed away, zipped up our pants, and walked over to the wash basins. Even though we were wearing name badges, they wouldn't have been necessary since we quickly identified with each other. We had a class together in our junior year. He said,

"Let's take a little walk outside; I have something I'd like to talk to you about." We sauntered out into the parking lot.

My new-found friend told me he is an attorney, a senior partner in the city's largest and most successful law firm. I told him, in a nutshell, what I do and the things I have been involved in through the years. He said, "I think you and I may have a common affinity." Then he said, "Oh hell, I'm not going to beat around the bush about it—I'm bisexual." I said, "I had a hunch we're both gay." At that point he looked much relieved—the speculation was gone. He said, "I guess there's nothing we can do about it here and now." If it had been seven or eight years earlier, I would have suggested we go to one of the darker reaches of the parking area and I would have "gone down" on him then and there between the parked cars. However, the curse of AIDS has put the fear of God in me. I don't want to take a chance on Him letting me down.

My legal friend told me that after two years of marriage, his first wife confessed that she was a lesbian and that she had no business being married to him, particularly since he wanted a family and she didn't. Even though she too was bisexual, he never let her know of his gay status. He had now been married to the same woman for thirty-one years and they had a son and two daughters and three grandkids. It was obvious, from the discussion, he was proud of his family, including his wife who had no knowledge of his bisexuality.

My friend suggested that we plan on getting together one of these days, even though his hometown is about two hours from where I presently live. He said he had a convenient rendezvous place. All I had to do was let him know a few hours in advance of my arrival. He gave me one of his business cards with his office phone number on it and said, "I'll make myself available for two or three hours, providing I'm not in court, and we'll have some gratifying fun together."

The following evening, at home, we were browsing through

Sue's graduation yearbook. There were several pictures of my legal friend. I discovered he was captain of one of the varsity teams in his senior year. Alongside one of his pictures was his signature with the notation above: "Good luck, Sue, in the years ahead. Your happy face was an inspiration to me." I asked Sue whether she remembered so-and-so. She said, "Do I! He was quite a ladies man; couldn't keep his hands off the girls." "Really," I prompted. "I should know," she responded, "I had two classes with him, Spanish and United States History, and we both served on a committee of CSF [California Scholarship Federation]."

At the reunion, Sue and I got recognition for being married the longest. When our names were called, the band struck up strains of "I Want A Girl Just Like The Girl That Married Dear Ole Dad." We were depicted as the couple having the most enduring relationship. I enjoyed the recognition but felt guilt about what I was being distinguished for. Through the years I have been perceived as the good guy, but if the real me were ever disclosed, in all probability I would be the bad guy.

When I was president of my own food-products distribution corporation in Southern California, my son sometimes worked for me on his summers off from college. One afternoon in my office we were reminiscing over some of the good times of the past and the present prosperity of the business when Mark made a comment I will always cherish. He said, "Dad, you're one hell of a man." It was obvious, in spite of my inward psychological temperament, I portrayed the enviable image of an admirable role model to him.

My wife has always been a good sport, in more ways than one. Even though she isn't the outdoor-girl type, all our married life Sue has tried to keep pace with me in many vigorous sporting activities. In 1984, we hiked together to the top of Half Dome in Yosemite National Park. For the first half of the day we rode mules from the stables on the floor of the valley to the base on the back side of the Dome. The rocky mountainside trail was precarious at times even for the sure-footed animals. When we reached the base of the Dome we started our climb straight up the cable foot trail to the top, stopping a number of times to catch our breath and to rest a few minutes. It was an exhausting experience, much more so for Sue. But when we got to the top, the majestic view made it all worthwhile.

It was a crisp, clear summer day and we could see about twenty miles in all directions. Sue said, "I feel so much closer to God." The large circular swimming pool, perhaps sixty-five to seventy-five feet across, at the renowned Ahwahnee Hotel on the floor of the valley below appeared about the size of a blue dime. In the eyes of God we must have looked like two tiny grains of sand that drifted on to the magnificent, formidable rock. Sixteen years earlier I had made the climb with our young son Mark, but there was something special about this—it was just Sue and I together.

Today, I have a culpable feeling about the way I have, or more properly stated, haven't treated Sue through the years. She deserves so much more caring affection than she has gotten from me. She has always been enthusiastic about pleasing me, in every way she can. For example, she is a connoisseur's cook and methodically plans her menus around my likes and dislikes.

But psychologically, we are two diverse personalities—she moral and virtuous, me loose and licentious. In the bedroom, we have little in common, and there are times, for months on end, when we go without sex altogether. I won't force myself on her. For sure, she is one wife who has never been raped by her husband.

Nonetheless, my demeanor and image around home and with our friends is the epitome of honorable. I suppose that's due, in part, to the longevity of our marriage. Most people think Sue and I are the exemplary model of married life. What they don't know is best for all concerned.

6

Role of the Gay in Everyday Life

If all the gays were to vanish from the face of the earth, this would be a pretty sad place. Some of the greatest and most notable talents and intellects in this world are gay. Through the centuries homosexuality has been found in royalty, nobility, and all levels of the social classes. They're all around us, and our lives and well-being depend on many of them.

In World War II, the military services were abounding with homosexuals, both male and female. The WACS and WAVES particularly were infiltrated with lesbians. It was a way of life that appealed to many of them. Uncle Sam needed all the young men he could get, and if you didn't arrive at the induction center in "drag," you were in. Homosexual activities flourished, almost unrestrained, in the army, navy, and Marine Corps in those days. Undoubtedly, it was due, to a large degree, to men living with men and women living with women, often in very close quarters. The homos and bis loved it. Then, there were those straight cads who feigned homosexuality in order to get a Section 8 (undesirable) discharge. A recent spoof of this type was Corporal Maxwell Klinger on TV's "M*A*S*H." Many of them succeeded, only to find the scam backfired. They were blackballed from getting responsible jobs for years to come, especially in the federal government. Of course, all that has changed today with nondiscrimination and human rights protection.

After World War II and in the early 1950s, Uncle Sam decided he didn't want those people on his payroll any longer—people who had put their hearts into winning the war. The witch hunts of Senator Joe McCarthy were not only looking for Communists in federal government positions, but homosexuals as well. The war was over and now homosexuals were considered to be subversives. The unjustifiable contention was that the Soviets were penetrating the ranks of top security government personnel and coercing homosexuals, through blackmail, to become Soviet spies. Gays were harassed with police entrapment. Gays in federal jobs were particularly vulnerable and constantly persecuted. If you were discovered to be homosexual, your employment would be terminated with loss of all accrued retirement benefits. This was an annihilating blow to loyal, longtime civil servants.

At about this time the gay liberation movement was developing. Forty years ago the slang term for homosexual was queer. The organized homosexuals in the underground movement detested the word queer and wanted a more apropos moniker. In selecting a replacement for the degrading word queer, the strategy was to come up with a name that would create a whole new image for homosexuals and lesbians. And, now more than forty years later we find the name took and stuck. It's no longer a queer world, it's the gay culture.

It was only twenty-five or thirty years ago that Negros, as they were called then, were violently persecuted in this country. They were not openly accepted in our social circles. It was strictly a matter of social bigotry, although commonly referred to as racism. The bigots called them "niggers" and eventually the words Negro and "nigger" were replaced with black. Today, black is beautiful. It's been a long hard pull, but blacks have "arrived," and they hold some of the most enviable, influential, and powerful positions in our society.

Gays have long been discriminated against because of their sexual preference, just as blacks had been the target of biased bigotry because of their ethnic heritage. We are both minorities. I suppose life could be worse—I could be a black gay. I'm really only kidding about this because I've known a couple of blacks gays, who were outstanding human beings. Perhaps gays are on their way to being openly accepted in our society just as blacks are today.

It wasn't so many years ago that if homosexuals were caught in the act of doing their "thing," it was an offense for which they could just about be hanged. The resulting incarceration and humiliation, with its ruinous results, would almost make them wish they had been hanged. In the past ten to fifteen years, courts and legal jurisdictions have become compassionate in dealing with matters relating to homosexuality. It seems now that homosexuality is legally sanctioned, providing you are a consenting adult doing your "thing" in privacy. Could it be that today homosexuality has infiltrated the ranks of law enforcement and there are gay district attorneys and gay judges sitting on the bench, passing sentences and administering justice in matters relating to homosexuality? In any case, a trend of sympathy has developed for the plight of the gay person in just the last few years. This may not be true in the thinking of Jerry Falwell and Anita Bryant, but it is so with millions of other Americans. Gays have become a strong force in the political arena. Their strength has been a powerful factor in changing legislation in many states, especially in regard to job discrimination. It's ironic that now Washington, D.C., has the second largest concentration of gays in the nation, second only to San Francisco. There are compelling reasons to believe homosexuality is not uncommon in the law-making bodies of our government. The archives of the *Washington Post* attest to this, e.g., members of Congress having sexual relations with male pages of the House and Senate.

So, what else is new? Really, it's old hat. There has to be a lot of gays in government today, both in elected and civil service positions. The gay-rights movement has had its impact.

What is a gay? Who is gay? Gays are people we rely on for our everyday way of life; they're in every career, occupation, vocation, profession, and work. Gays are bankers, stevedores, attorneys, professional athletes, CPAs, ministers, truck drivers, doctors, engineers, ditch diggers, judges, business owners, factory workers, plumbers, housewives, corporate presidents, teachers, police officers, nurses, electricians, salesmen, secretaries, public and government officials, and on and on. And, most of them are "closet" gays who have their own secret, discreet contacts and relationships. In gay parlance, men who conceal their gay status are known as "closet queens." "Closet" denotes secretive actions and associations. A "closet queen" may be anyone from your parish priest to the guy next door—the father of five kids, whom everyone thinks is the exemplification of family life.

Then, how do you spot a gay? You don't! Gays come in both sexes, all sizes and colors, and represent every ethnic background, nationality, socioeconomic level, religion, and political viewpoint. Sexual orientation, religion, and politics have nothing to do with one another. I, for example, am both a liberal, hypersexual gay and a Roman Catholic, conservative Republican. Believe it or not, even I like Rush Limbaugh, that gay-bashing, wacko-conservative, network-radio talk-show host. Some of the most respected and influential men and women in their respective communities are homosexual or bisexual. God in His infinite wisdom came up with different strokes for different folks. But who is to decide which of us is different?

New York's celebrated Gay Men's Chorus includes doctors, lawyers, professors, and business executives. In ten years the group has grown to 136 talented men and has won critical acclaim. The chorus appears annually in a sold-out concert at Carnegie Hall. Even though new men are continually joining the group, its growth is not that noticeable due to the loss of members to AIDS. The AIDS pandemic has taken the lives of 37 members of the chorus.

One of the more notable gays was the late Malcolm Forbes, the multimillionaire business and finance publisher. He was an exuberant sportsman, cosmopolitan, and an unabashed bon vivant. In 1989 he hosted a $2 million seventieth birthday celebration for himself in Tangier, Morocco. Forbes paid for air fare and accommodations for all his invited guests.

About twenty years ago I was aboard Malcolm Forbes's multimillion-dollar yacht, "The Highlander." It was tied up at Jack London Square in Oakland, California. I was in a small group that was taken on a tour of the boat by its skipper. Included in that group were the mayor of Oakland and the president of the Oakland Port Commission. We didn't have the pleasure of meeting Forbes; he was across the bay in San Francisco that afternoon. After learning that Forbes was gay, I have often thought that his magnificent boat may have been used at times as the rendezvous place of floating orgies.

Another notable gay was the late maestro Leonard Bernstein, laureate director of the New York Philharmonic Orchestra. He was a conductor, composer, and pianist, and one of the greatest musicians of our time. He composed a number of resplendent symphonies, including "The Age of Anxiety." In his earlier years, Bernstein openly led a licentious gay life. Throughout his career he surrounded himself with handsome young men, many of whom were protégés. As his brilliance became known in the music world and his reputation grew, his critics turned to fans and his sexual orientation was forgotten about.

Both Leonard Bernstein and Malcolm Forbes died in 1990— Forbes a short time after his lavish, much-publicized birthday party in Morocco; perhaps it was his swan song.

Many celebrity male bisexuals attempt to conceal their gay orientation and to portray a heterosexual image by surrounding themselves with females for conspicuous occasions. Elizabeth Taylor was a frequent companion of Malcolm Forbes in the years prior to his death. She was Forbes's hostess for many of his social functions, including the pompous birthday celebration in Morocco. There were rumors that she and Forbes planned to be married. For many years Merv Griffin has had Eva Gabor at his side for most public appearances. For nine years Eva has been his "front lady," telling the media that she and Merv are engaged.

I get confused when I see a guy wearing an earring in a pierced ear. Many people come to the immediate conclusion, when seeing a male wearing an earring, that the guy is gay. This is only an assumption. However, an earring on a gay usually has a significant implication. In many gay circles, an earring, depending on which ear it is worn, indicates the guy is spoken for or is involved in a monogamous gay relationship. On the other hand, it may be a young man who just wants to wear one of mama's earrings now and then. There are many types of earrings worn by some gays, including ornate danglers. However, the more discreet gay may wear a tiny diamond chip. Gays have to be cautious about approaching another guy with an earring in a pierced ear. Sometimes the other guy is a straight cad bent on gay bashing and the earring is a lure for the unsuspecting.

With the genesis of "women's lib," the time-honored image of the American woman in the work force has been tarnished. She is no longer looked upon as the sweet, tender, weaker sex that needs guidance and protection. Many women have become macho females as a result of their combative, competitive zeal. I'm still old fashioned and chivalrous enough that I believe women deserve to be treated differently from men. When a woman enters a room, I will come to my feet; I will open the door for her and pull out her chair. There is something special about women. None of us would be here if it were not for a woman.

Two men can make love with each other, but neither can produce another human being.

Too many women are trying to imitate and compete totally with their male peers in the work environment, not just in knowledge and perception, but also in physical characteristics and proficiency. Somehow, I just can't believe they're all lesbians. A few months ago I happened to see an equipment installer and at first glance I said to myself, there's something strange about that guy. At second glance, it turned out to be a woman and not the type I'd want to wake up with in bed in the morning. There are similar types in executive, professional, and office positions and undoubtedly many are lesbians. I'm so glad all females in the business world are not "women's libbers." Bisexuality in some respects is incredible—the best of two worlds. However, I like manly men and feminine women. This would be a pretty dull life sexually and otherwise, if we were all neuters.

When I was a young man, we never heard of such a thing as date rape; either it was a date or it was rape. If a young lady let a man go that far, she was a consenting adult or a victim of her own indiscretion. In this era of women's lib and feminist activists, a man has to be extremely cautious about how he compliments a woman in the workplace. It could be interpreted as sexual harassment. An extreme example was the agonizing human drama of the Clarence Thomas Senate hearings, in which a female and male black were pitted against each other by powerful, influential white men. This televised circus was a corrupt, damaging travesty of the process with lasting implications. I can't conceivably believe that sexual harassment could ever be classified as a criminal offense. Whether or not it is a crime will always be a matter of the sensitive perception and attitude of the parties involved. Millions of happy marriages started with so-called sexual harassment. I suppose any man with a wife could be perceived as being guilty of sexual harassment.

The Justice Thomas confirmation fiasco should have put all

men on notice to keep their distance from women, particularly in the work environment. You never know who has conniving designs on you. If a man has sexual inclinations toward a pretty female, he's only a normal human being. But men are becoming paranoid about sexual harassment, even with the ones they think they know so well. Such a philosophical mind-set could surely foster the spread of homosexuality.

When certain straight people learn there is a gay in their midst, they have a trauma. A wife may feel her husband is in jeopardy. A father may feel his children are at risk. Many people seem to have the idea that homosexuals zero in on minors and young people. I don't understand this. Gays are no worse or better than straights when it comes to morality. If a fifty-year-old heterosexual man is bent on extracurricular sexual activities, he won't be attracted to sixty- and seventy-year-old women. Let's face it, in all probability, he'll be zeroing in on twenty-five- and thirty-five-year-old women. If he's the "dirty old man" type, it might be eighteen- and nineteen-year-old girls, and this is not uncommon. Some people seem to think there is such a difference in the ethics and morality of homosexuals. I have known heterosexual men who were extremely indiscriminate and promiscuous and much more sexually active than I have ever been. I think I have known a few heterosexual ladies that fall into this same category.

A few years ago I read a magazine article about an NFL quarterback, a national hero at the time. He was boasting about having had intercourse with more than two hundred different women in a period of one year. He must have used the "bench mark" system and even had it categorized by age group. He preferred "very young" females. He's a celebrity today and whenever I hear his name or see his face in print or on television, I think of that article.

I believe most gays have a person l code of moral and social ethics that rules their conscience. Parents have no need to fear for their children's well-being when gays are present any more than they would when the average straight person is with them. There are innumerable cases of heterosexuals being convicted of child molestation, many times more often than homosexuals being convicted of the same crime. However, when a gay person is convicted of child molestation, the righteous, honorable moralists will say, "I told you so."

I have never had the slightest desire to have any kind of sexual contact with children, perhaps young adults, nineteen or twenty years old in certain circumstances, but never minors. I can't imagine myself even discussing sex in any form with any of my grandchildren. It was awkward and ticklish enough trying to explain "the birds and the bees" to my own son when he was ten or twelve years old. And I remember my wife went through the same thing with our young daughter when she started menstruating.

Sometime ago a gay acquaintance told me his fourteen-year-old grandson had recently gotten braces on his teeth. He said the boy told him how difficult it was now having oral copulation. He said he (his grandson) had sex with both boys and girls. I registered a look of shock, not only about the young boy's sexual prowess, but also his grandfather discussing it with him. The guy assured me he wouldn't think of touching the boy sexually. He said, however, the boy confided in him and they often had intimate discussions about sex.

Why does there have to be such a disparaging attitude toward gays? If you learned at the zero hour that the surgeon about to save your life was gay, would you call off the operation? If the only attorney in a law firm capable of successfully defending you in a law suit was gay, would you select another? Narrow-mindedness could cost you your life or possibly a fortune. What difference does it make about the doctor's or lawyer's private and personal life? He may be a Republican and you a Democrat, or he may be a Jew and you a Protestant or Catholic.

So what? He has a code of professional ethics he is sworn to and he's going to do the very best for you he knows how and possibly can, regardless of the fact that he is homosexual and you are heterosexual. And he probably couldn't care less about your sexual preferences.

Donald J. Trump, New York's whiz-kid financial and business entrepreneur, in the early stages of amassing his fortune retained the late Roy Cohn as his attorney. Trump knew Cohn was homosexual, as did numerous other people in the business world. Nevertheless, Trump had great admiration for Cohn's law brilliance and considered him not only a business associate, but also a personal friend. Cohn had many personal friends in influential places, including Nancy Reagan.

Recently the famed Chippendales male burlesque troupe came to our city for a two-performance, one-night stand. Two of my wife's good friends wanted to see the show and talked Sue into going along. At the zero hour, the husband of one of Sue's friends decided it was not a proper place for his wife to be seen in and she bowed out. As prudish as Sue is, she is not adverse to being entertained by a little buffoonery. She persuaded me into going along with her and her friend. They believed they would feel better about the whole thing if they were in the company of a male escort.

The first eight or ten rows in front of the stage were packed with young ladies in the age range, I would guess, from eighteen to thirty-five. In the last six or eight rows, which we were in, you saw older sophisticated ladies, including what appeared to be a number of grandmothers. And there were a number of men throughout the audience. I couldn't let Sue know my evaluation of the performers, but the seven young men in the show were gorgeous "hunks" of masculinity—beautiful specimens with statuesque physiques. Due to my sexual orientation, I have an uncanny knack for recognizing homosexuals. It was obvious to me, that at least four of the seven guys in the show were gay; it was hard to believe they all weren't. I'm not so sure their talents would not have been even more appreciated by an audience of gay men, rather than a small army of hot and horny straight females.

In their diverse acts, the guys in the show peeled it down to just a hair short of exposing the very best. The lustful women in the audience went wild, squealing and yelling with frenzied ecstasy. One of the real eye-catchers was a guy about twenty-three to perhaps twenty-seven years old. He was a beautiful six-foot bronze-skinned Adonis with locks of dark hair and a sparkling diamond on the lobe of his left ear. There was another area of his body that sparkled and stood out also, although it wasn't as totally visible as the ear lobe with the diamond.

At the conclusion of each performer's act, he would go down to the front of the stage where eager, lecherous females in their wild, excited state were clamoring for their turn to kiss the guy. Each would give him some folded money (assumed to be a dollar bill) for the privilege. The guy was in his scant G-string and the girls and ladies were obsessed with touching him, if only on the face or shoulder. I thought at the time, if the guys really were gay, they must be laughing up the proverbial sleeve at all those harebrained women who paid $25 just to get in. There had to be at least seventy-five to one hundred women who paid to kiss those studs after their acts, and it was something more than just a smooch on the cheek. I zeroed in on one young woman in the audience who made five trips to the stage and kissed five different performers. It's hard to believe I may have been jealous or envious, but anything's possible.

At the end of the show there was a photo session and the women were given an opportunity to spend a few more bucks. They were invited up to the stage to have their picture taken with their favorite stud or studs in just his G-string. It was fun watching, since many of the ladies wanted their picture taken in an embrace with one or two of the guys together. When we left, there were a number of male vultures outside just waiting for the prey, which was now ripe and ready.

More Personal Experiences

When I was in business in Orange County, California, a number of my associates played golf one or two afternoons a week. Since I was not a golfer, I got my kicks and relaxation from spending two or three hours in the gay baths while my colleagues were out on the golf course. Besides sexual pleasure, these occasions gave me the opportunity of making new friends. One of the most interesting guys I met at the baths was "Phil." He was a career employee of the courts system of the State of California and held a responsible administrative position. It also turned out that we were Orange County neighbors and that he lived only about ten minutes from me. Our meeting at a gay bath on a summer afternoon in 1977 developed into an intimate seven-year friendship.

Phil lived in a beautiful home in a middle-income area. He had been married but was divorced when I met him. He had a sixteen-year-old son who lived with his mother half the time and with Phil the other half. Phil's wife knew he was gay, but their son did not. They had agreed in a pact that they would never tell him.

I had delightful, gratifying encounters with Phil at his home on the average of twice a month. On a half dozen occasions he came over to my house when Sue was out of town visiting our daughter or friends, but of course she never knew. My wife had heard me mention Phil on several occasions and understood he was a divorced professional I had met at our health club. I had told her, because of Phil's single status, he rarely got involved in social functions with married couples. I pretended that he was very hurt and bitter about his divorce and didn't enjoy fraternizing with married people, which was really a "crock." So, together, we never invited Phil to our home.

In the early summer of 1982, Phil told me he was planning a party for a number of gay friends on a Saturday night and would really like to have me involved. This posed a problem for me because of my wife. My gay sex life had been fairly easy to hide from her because my affairs were always during the day, when I was traveling, or when she was out of town. Occasionally I could fabricate an evening business meeting, but not on Saturday night. I had to concoct a story.

I told Sue that I had met Phil at the club and that he had invited me to join him and some guys on an overnight sailing excursion from Newport Beach to Catalina Island the following weekend. This was a logical story for me since I had owned a thirty-foot sloop and had long been a sailing enthusiast. I pretended that the guys were going to meet midday on Saturday and return late Sunday afternoon. This isn't the most ideal sailing schedule for such a long excursion, but Sue didn't question it. My wife thought the whole thing was great and told me I'd been working too hard and needed a little diversion. Little did she know, just how much diversion.

I arrived at Phil's early Saturday afternoon in very casual clothes, looking like I might be going on a sailing junket. A couple of Phil's friends were already on hand helping with preparations and I pitched in, too. The hub of the party activities was to be the garage. It was a three-car garage with the walls and ceiling finished off like a room of the house. One of the guys was hanging large poster type color photos of nudes, male and female. Phil had invited fifteen guys and three lesbians. An elaborate stereo system had already been set up in the garage for dancing. The other guy that was there was working on food items in the kitchen. I did various chores throughout the afternoon, including a couple of trips to a nearby supermarket. It was obvious a very lavish and sumptuous buffet was being put together. Then, at about five o'clock, a friend of Phil's arrived with several gourmet dishes. It turned out that he was not only a guest for the evening, but also a partner in a catering company. From there on, he took over preparation of the food and arrangement of the buffet in the dining room.

About six o'clock the guests began arriving and by seven most of them were there. Phil told me eleven of his male guests were homosexual and four, including him and me, were bisexual. He had also invited three lesbians. As the evening progressed there was a lot of dancing. Of course, men were dancing with men and the ladies with one another. This is something that has never appealed to me. As a matter of fact, a few years ago, I found it distasteful and disgusting. However, in my mellowing with age, I say, "To each his own." I was not the only wallflower; our host Phil and two or three of the other guys were also just watching.

This type of party was a first for me and very intriguing. There were so many meaningful glances and maneuvering, along with trendy conversation. I watched a couple of the guys leave the family room and go outside to the garden and disappear behind an elevated kiosk. They were gone about forty-five minutes. Then the three foxy ladies disappeared for more than an hour. I saw them come down the stairs, one at a time about five minutes apart. I'm sure they thought they were being crafty, but it wasn't hard to guess that they must have been in an upstairs bedroom having a little threesome orgy. Phil had not intended for his party to be a disreputable social affair and it was not. The guests were well behaved and extremely considerate of their host.

The party began to disperse about one o'clock in the morning. Phil had asked two of his other friends if they would like to stay overnight. They accepted his invitation and by two o'clock the four of us were the only guests remaining. Now, the party really began. We had an all-night orgy that wouldn't seem to stop. By nine o'clock Sunday morning I was devastated, completely wrung out. I told Phil I just had to have a few hours sleep before going home. It was at about this time that his other two friends left. Phil and I went to bed and slept till two o'clock in the afternoon.

In gay parlance, Phil was known as a "size queen." A size queen is a gay who is attracted to and prefers men that are heavy hung with large genitals. Size queens are not necessarily well endowed themselves; however, Phil was and obviously his intimate friends were too.

When I arrived home about four o'clock, Sue said, "You look like you've had a workout; you must have run into some foul weather." I said, "We did, a few miles out yesterday and had to turn back. We didn't get back until long after dark and then only as far as Huntington Beach." I told her that we dropped anchor there overnight and sailed back to Newport that day. Again, I had that big guilt feeling. I felt I should get the award of the year from the "Liars Club of America." Nevertheless, it was two days I'll never forget.

During the last couple of years that we lived in Orange County, I got very much involved with two ladies who were good friends of both my wife and me. I suppose you'd say they were family friends. One I will call "Linda"; she was three years younger than I. The other, "Barbara," was nineteen years younger. Barbara and Linda were also mutual friends, so we all knew one another.

Linda worked in the accounting office of a large corporation. Barbara worked for a travel agency. Both were very attractive and charming ladies. Linda was a well-endowed, buxom widow with a curvaceous body. Barbara was a svelte, suave young divorcee. They both lived in apartments in the same complex, within sight of each other. When my wife and I first went to Orange County, we lived in the same complex for two years.

On several occasions after we moved into our own home, Sue had Linda over for dinner. A number of times I caught her looking intently at my crotch. For some reason many women can't take their eyes off a man's crotch. They're really curious about the "monster" that lurks beind the zipper. Linda and I seemed to have connecting vibes. She probably caught me gazing at her voluptuous bosom. At any rate, through a series of events, I found myself in Linda's apartment one evening when my wife was out of town, two hundred miles away, visiting relatives. We had just arrived back at her apartment after a pleasurable dining experience. When we got in the door, Linda put one arm around my neck and with the other hand pulled down the zipper on my pants. She really did want to see what was behind that zipper. I didn't disappoint her, since I had a hard erection on its way. Soon we were undressing each other.

Linda had a beautiful body. She truly was a sensuous, voluptuous woman, not fat or even plump; there was just so much to play with. The next thing I knew, we were on her waterbed and I was down on her doing the oral bit. Soon, she decided she wanted her share and we were in the 69 position. After a while, we deecided we wanted a firmer surface and adjourned to the living room floor. While on the floor, I learned that Linda liked anal intercourse just as well as vaginal intercourse. Even though she had had a hysterectomy, it seemed that she enjoyed anal sex almost more than vaginal. I stayed for the night. From the time we got back from dinner in the evening until the following morning, I had three orgasms—one oral, one vaginal, and one anal. If variety is truly the spice of life, that was one of the spiciest nights I have ever lived. That lady really brought out the beast in me.

About a month later, and again through a series of events, I found myself taking Barbara out to dinner. Sue was gone for three days visiting our daughter and family, about five hours away. When we returned to Barbara's apartment, we had barely gotten in the door when we were locked in an embrace. Then, I was raising her dress and pulling down her pantyhose while she was unbuttoning her blouse. In less than five minutes we were both naked. Before the night was over I realized Barbara had a ravaging appetite for sex. She was even more of a nympho-maniac than Linda, although she didn't like anal intercourse. I left early the following morning.

A week later, I called Linda on the phone when I was in my office in the evening. She came right to the point: "What have you got going with Barbara?" I pretended innocence: "What do you mean?" She told me that she had seen me coming out of Barbara's apartment one morning. I simply responded that I believed in sharing the wealth and then suggested a three-some next Saturday. Linda said, "That's O.K. with me, but I won't be the instigator. Barbara is young enough to be my daughter." I told her I was sure I could arrange it.

To make a long story short, the following Saturday after-noon we had a stupendous four-hour three-way orgy in Barbara's apartment. If I went into explicit detail, the moralists would call it degenerate, so I will spare them the revelation. I had told Sue that I would be at an all-day business seminar on Satur-day, and it was the most stimulating "seminar" I ever attended. I believe if my wife ever learned about this, my life would be in jeopardy. As a matter of fact, Sue would kill me if she ever found out about a lot of things. I sometimes think of her as one of the holier-than-thou moralists, the same girl I slept with in hotels and motels before we were married. Perhaps she wanted me at any price.

That orgy with two such beautiful and sensual ladies was the first of some of the greatest sexual experiences in my life and there were several more with the same cast in the next few months. The ladies were obviously straight and didn't have the slightest suspicion of my bisexuality. They were utterly captivated and delighted with my virile performance and endurance. Then, too, I'm very well endowed. I thought to myself, all this in spite of the aging process; yet I have to admit, there were times in those orgies with Barbara and Linda that the thought crossed my mind—what a way to die!

As far as the aging process is concerned, I believe age is a state of mind. My mind tells me that I want to and can do the things I did in my youth; so I refuse to grow old physically and mentally and really believe that I'm indestructible. Sure, I have a few gray hairs and I'm not the jock I was even ten years ago, but I'm working at it. I somehow feel I'll be a stud at age eighty, if God is compassionate enough to let me live that long. It's all a matter of attitude. As they say, I'm not getting older; I'm getting better. When you're over the hill, you pick up speed.

I have often thought that one of the most exciting and gratifying sexual experiences would be an orgy with two compatible bisexual couples—two males and two females. No holds barred—males for females, females for males, males for males, and females for females. From my perspective as a bisexual, this would be the ultimate, all-encompassing utopia. I'm sure such orgies are common practice with certain people. I have seen movies of them and nothing is left to the lusty imagination.

I would like to get more involved with women, but there are too many considerations and inducements—candy, flowers, perfume, little boutique gifts, the dining experience, and on and on, all this hopefully leading up to a sexual encounter. When two men get together with sex as the objective, there aren't all the ulterior, attentive, solicitous frills. Men have only one thing in mind and that's the orgasm and foreplay that leads up to it. If the other guy is clean and attractive, my main concern is whether or not he is discreet and I consider him safe. I'm only interested in one thing and that's his body. A man doesn't usually care whether or not another man is married. Women want to get more involved and this presents a serious problem to a man who has no intention of leaving his wife. Whether gay or straight, most men are just different from women when it comes to sex. Men have an instinctive, natural freedom about sex. The gay baths were a good example of male sexual freedom, although I have seen some tender, timid individuals in the steam rooms who wouldn't uncross their legs.

During the time I was in business in Orange County, I received an invitation, for both my wife and me, to join an exclusive little social group. It consisted of fourteen married couples in the age range of forty to fifty-five. They referred to themselves as the "key set." The group was made up of small-business owners, corporate executives, and professional people, including a banker and two physicians. I knew three members of the group who also knew my wife. On the last Saturday of each month the group would meet early in the evening for cocktails at the home of one of the couples. When they arrived, the husband would put his car keys in a bowl on a table. After an hour or two, when the party was breaking up, each of the ladies would select a set of keys from the bowl. The owner of the keys was her date for the evening, the guy she would go home with after dinner at one of Orange County's many fine restaurants. I was told that the ladies could identify their own husband's keys and that couples who had kids at home would farm them out for the weekend or, if this wasn't convenient, the guy would take his date to a hotel or motel. It was the classic wife-swapping scheme. The whole thing sounded fantastic to me, but I never have told my wife about the invitation. I had a feeling that if she found out I would even entertain such an idea, it could cause problems. It would go over like a lead balloon with Sue. She is just too much internalized due to her puritanical upbringing.

While living in Orange County, my wife and I maintained a membership in a superlative health club. It was a huge, modern facility with about 4,000 members, including men and women. There were private sections for men and women, as well as common areas. In the private men's sections, men could use the sauna, steam room, and spa in the nude, as in most health clubs. If there is a means of dispelling the myth "all men are created equal," it is in the private men's sections of health clubs.

One evening in the autumn of 1982, I was sitting in the large spa with three or four other guys. Soon, all had left except one young man. He was sitting about three feet away and we began talking about how soothing the penetrating, bubbling hot water was coming out of the jets. As we were talking, he was inching close to me. Soon he was only about a foot away. I probably would have moved, except there was no one else in the spa. When he put his hand on my leg, my penis began to stand up. I reached over and touched his and it was already stiff as a rod. Before I knew it, we were sitting there stroking each other under the water. If someone had come in, they couldn't have seen what we were doing, but sitting as close as we were looked awfully suspicious. I told him we had to stop before we were caught, so we moved apart. It was just in the nick of time, for within the next three or four minutes there were five more guys in the spa.

Since our erections were pretty stiff, we had to remain in the water for a few minutes before we could get out. My friend left the spa first and motioned me to follow him to the showers. In the showers, I got the chance to admire his body. He was a handsome, blue-eyed blond with a gorgeous, light hairy masculine body. He was well hung, which I had obviously detected under the water. After showering, we headed for our lockers and agreed to meet in the lobby.

In the lobby, my new chum introduced himself as Steve. Steve told me he was nineteen years old and a premed student at the neighboring University of California at Irvine. He said he lived with his parents, brother, and sister in nearby Newport Beach. His father was an M.D. Steve too was bisexual, having a couple of girlfriends and a couple of boyfriends. I told him a little about myself, that I was president of a small corporation and also lived nearby. Steve motioned to his van over in the parking lot and invited me inside.

When we got into the van, Steve locked the doors from the inside. The van was outfitted with deep-pile carpeting from behind the front seats to the rear doors. Within a blink of an eye we were on the carpet taking our clothes off, and soon we were in the 69 position oral copulating. Steve and I went at it off and on for about an hour. Since we had just showered, we tongued each other's anus (in gay jargon, this is called "rimming"). For those who don't know, contact with two such sensitive and responsive parts of the body as the tongue and anus creates an ecstatic sensation for both parties. With many lesbians, it's as much enjoyed in the overall sexual experience as cunnilingus. We both had orgasms. No one knew we were there, since the van was also outfitted with smoked one-way glass and you couldn't see in from the outside.

In the next few months, Steve and I had five more encounters. On our third meeting, Steve told me that it was amazing that we hit it off so well considering our age span. I said, "Remember, Steve, the best music is played on old instruments."

Early one afternoon in the spring of 1983, I left my office in Santa Ana, Orange County, and drove to a gay bath in Long Beach. It wasn't a long drive and I was a frequent customer. As I was checking in, a guy I had seen there on several occasions also came in. He was about my age and his clothes obviously reflected the status of a professional or a businessman. He was impeccably dressed with a charcoal gray, pin-striped suit, brightly shined shoes, crisp white shirt, and an expensive-looking tie. He was a handsome dude. About a half hour later I walked past his room, looked into the open door, and saw that he was lying naked on his stomach on the bed. This was an indication that he wanted anal intercourse. I went down the hall a bit and continued walking while I was thinking about it. I have always been very discreet and cautious about anal intercourse. Because of my apprehension about health considerations, anal intercourse has been an insignificant part of my gay sex life, although I love it from the aggressor's standpoint. This guy looked as pure as a breeze off the ocean, so I walked into his room. We talked a few minutes, then he pulled my wrapper off, checked me out, and said, "Let's do it." I was with him only about ten to fifteen minutes. After that, I made a beeline for the urinals and showers.

Six days after the anal encounter, I got out of bed early in the morning and couldn't urinate. I discovered pus, about the consistency of toothpaste, oozing out of my penis. I was horrified since Sue was so close at hand. In spite of our sexual mismatch, we have always slept together in the same bed. After breakfast, I was able to get out of the house without her noticing anything peculiar.

I was reluctant to go to the family physician, but came to the conclusion I had to. When I got to my office I called for an appointment. The nurse told me the doctor could see me at two o'clock that afternoon. Those were anguishing hours between the time I called and the time I saw the doctor. I had never had anything like that before and never since.

The doctor examined me and immediately said I had gonorrhea. I told him that I had gotten it from a young lady employed by one of my business associates, after an office party. The doctor prescribed a massive dose of penicillin, which he said would be effective immediately; luckily it was. He also gave me the same prescription for Sue because I was worried that I might have passed it on to her. The only problem was what I was going to tell her. Once again, I had to concoct a story.

I went home early that afternoon and told Sue that I had just come from the doctor because I had been suffering from painful urination the past two or three days. I pretended that the doctor diagnosed my condition as a urinary infection and gave me the same prescription for her just in case I had passed it on to her. She didn't question my story and took her medication. I thanked God I was off the hook, but I did sweat it out for a few hours. That was the last time I had anal intercourse with anyone. It was about then that the whole world was becoming aware of the deadly disease AIDS.

About this time, a lot of things began going wrong in my life. Our business, which my wife and I had built from scratch and after eight years had sales of $3 million a year, was about to collapse. We were in Chapter XI Bankruptcy, not due to insolvency but because of my poor judgment in contractual negotiations. We had twelve dedicated employees and the company was estimated to be worth $1 million. Eventually we lost not only the business, but our home as well. It was total ruination, just at a time when we thought we were on our way to a future of financial independence and affluence. As we look back now, we can't imagine how we maintained our sanity.

At this point, my drinking had gotten out of hand. One Sunday afternoon, a week after the gonorrhea episode, I was arrested for drunk driving less than six blocks from our home. I had gone to a nearby hardware store to get a couple of items for a household project I was working on. One officer stopped me and then he called for another officer. They were a little indecisive about taking me to jail, but finally decided to do so and I was taken away in handcuffs. My car was impounded, and my poor, dear, distraught wife, who was working in her rose garden, saw my car go by our home on the back of a tow truck. At the jail, I was subjected to a urine test, fingerprinting, being booked, and an incarceration of five hours. Sue was waiting for me when I was released. This happened before the California drunk driving laws became so severely stringent. Nevertheless, this little incident cost me $1,100. Because of the borderline situation my attorney, through plea bargaining, was able to get the charge reduced from drunk driving to exhibition driving and the fine reduced from $500 to $350. His fee was $750.

I was very bitter about the drunk driving arrest, but it may be one of the best things that ever happened to me. I needed my wings clipped. There were times I'd drive away from a business luncheon after having three or four martinis. A partner in the law firm that handled my bankruptcy told me the same thing happened to him about two years before. He said his arrest had been a timely deterrent toward his becoming a hopeless alcoholic. He said it also probably prevented him from killing someone, including himself, because when he had a snoot full, he drove with reckless abandon. I was just the opposite. When I knew I had too much to drink, I drove with extreme caution and that's how I was spotted.

Other than bankruptcy, the arrest for drunk driving was the most disparaging, humiliating experience in all my life. Even though the charge was reduced from drunk driving for the record, I was on conditional probation for three years. Bankruptcy, venereal disease, and drunk driving—I felt like a criminal. This was my lowest time ever, and my self-esteem had sunk to the point where I felt I'd have to reach up to touch bottom. It was difficult to believe at that time there would ever be a new beginning, but God has been good to me.

After the sad misfortunes of 1983, including the loss of our home, we decided to leave Southern California and return to the San

Joaquin Valley. Since I had completely divorced myself from the gay baths, I found and utilized a new approach for making contact with other desirable gays. It's *The Advocate,* the most widely circulated gay publication in the entire country.

It is a biweekly magazine which boasts a readership of well in excess of 150,000. *The Advocate* was first published in 1967. In 1972 it had a paid circulation of nearly 35,000, and by 1986 that had risen to 81,604. A survey in the late 1970s showed that 70 percent of *The Advocate's* readers had college degrees with 9 percent of those having doctoral degrees, and 35 percent of the total readership having annual incomes in excess of $25,000 at that time. Half the readers contributed to a political campaign in the year just prior to the survey, and 83 percent reported having voted in the last election. Today, the publication is available on numerous newsstands and by subscription. It is also found in the periodical and newspaper section of some public libraries.

The Advocate is recognized for its credible news coverage and unbiased editorials, and its classified ad section is a great meeting place for gays. Secretly, I maintain a post office box and have advertised twice in the past four years to make contact with prudent, discreet gays in my area. Since I'm a "closet" gay and can't attend gay parties and functions or patronize the bars, this has proved to be a great way for me to maintain contact with the gay world. I have been able to exercise maximum caution and discretion in personally meeting the contacts I have made, and the results of my own ads as well as those I have answered have been rewarding. This is extremely important in my particular situation.

Today, and for the past three years, there are only two men with whom I have sexual relations. It's been a bountiful bisexual life, but now with the stark reality of AIDS it's down to only two. One I will call Carl, because that is one of his names. The other I will refer to as Dr. Bob. Both are handsome bisexuals and none of us has anything to do with anal intercourse; we're strictly interested in oral sex. I have sexual encounters with Carl at least once or twice a week. I get together with Bob about twice a month. Now that there is no such thing as safe sex anymore, one must have a tremendous confidence in his sexual partners. I have this confidence in Carl and Bob.

Dr. Bob is a Ph.D. and a state university professor. He is forty-four years old, divorced, and has a seventeen-year-old son. Bob comes from a well-to-do family. He and his son live in a fashionable home in an upper-income area. Bob's mother and father live on the family ranch about forty-five minutes away. His son spends a great deal of time with his grandparents on the ranch. Bob is at Stanford University three days a month as a guest lecturer. He has two lady friends and several boy-friends, and is on a constant social whirl. Bob is like a stud-horse in great demand.

Carl is the owner of a business that employs thirteen highly trained technicians. He is a workaholic, more so than myself. I'm the only one with whom he has any sexual relations at all and have been for some time. He is my age and has been married to the same woman for nearly as long as I have been married to my wife. They have a married daughter and two grandchild-ren, but from what Carl tells me, he and his wife haven't had sex with each other in eleven years. He says when they did, she would ask him, in the middle of intercourse, "Are you through yet?" He says it got to the point where he just couldn't bring himself to do it and finally didn't. It was almost two years since their last sex before she said anything about it. Despite his wife's complete lack of interest in sleeping with him, Carl is convinced that there is no other man and that his wife is not a lesbian. He says they love each other dearly, but only in a Platonic way as a child loves it parents. Neither Carl nor his wife are church-goers; however, they are very much involved in their social circles. I have pretty much come to the conclusion that for most men, if they don't get sex in one form, they'll get it in another.

When I first met Carl about four years ago, he told me the first time he ever got involved sexually with a man was just eight years before at the age of fifty-two. He said his wife would die if she had any inkling of his bisexual activities. Our rendezvous place is Carl's recreational vehicle, which he keeps in a private storage yard. It's really a land cruiser complete with shower and many luxuries and always ready to go with hot and cold running water. He keeps it in this standby condition, primarily for out-of-town guests and visiting relatives. It's more recreational than anyone knows. Carl and I meet there on an average of twice a week, depending on whether or not we're both in town. We've had some "sexsational" times in that RV.

One of the most enjoyable aspects of sex with Carl is the result of dental problems. When Carl was forty-seven, he had a ravaging periodontic disease. After several months of unsuccessful treatment, he finally had to have all his teeth extracted. Carl is a very handsome man and even though he wears dentures, you'd never suspect it. When we engage in oral copulation, he removes his false teeth. Minus teeth and with Carl's sensual exuberance, fellatio by him is a salacious sex experience. I sometimes almost wish I had no teeth and could reciprocate in the same way.

I have thought many times that one of the greatest advantages of being bisexual would be in my later years. Now that I have reached senior citizen status it's becoming more apparent each year that bisexuality does have advantages. I don't have quite the vigor and vitality I had twenty years ago. Nevertheless, I'm nowhere near losing my manly virility, but when that day comes, I'll still have an educated, palpitating tongue and a sensitive, receptive "oral cavity" (deep throat). Anyway, sooner or later all men are faced with the curse of impotency and when that occurs the oral aspects of bisexuality produce its greatest advantage.

Another erotic facet of my relationship with Carl is that he was never circumcised. His penis is long (seven inches) and thick, and the foreskin rarely comes all the way down over the head. It is exceptionally sensitive and responsive. All this makes him extremely hot and horny. Our oral encounters send him up the wall and many times he will have two orgasms to my one. I can't possibly comprehend how a woman could have lived with him for forty years and not have had sex with him in the past eleven of those forty. She has to be dead sexually. But, he still has a special kind of love for his wife and evidently she for him.

My wife, through an unusual set of circumstances, met Carl on an occasion when she was with me. She said, "I'll bet he and his wife would be a nice couple to know; why don't we try to cultivate a friendship with them?" It was a one-time meeting for her and the subject hasn't come up since. I don't think it would be such a good idea and Carl agrees.

My gay connections have all been sexual with no sincere attachments. Perhaps, in reality, I'm a "macho gay." However, many gay relationships revolve around emotional attachment, including affection, infatuation, devotion, and true love. There are even gay relationships where sex is absent—this has to be true love. Men do love men and women do love women. Although Platonic love among gays is not uncommon, for me it's not understandable. I can't seem to comprehend falling in love with a man and more so where no sexual gratification is involved. Nevertheless, most long-term, monogamous gay relationships do involve emotional love and fondness, whether sexual or Platonic.

I have been in love only once in my life. You will recall, I married my high school sweetheart. I'm sure that's the only love I've ever known, sexual or Platonic. Regardless of whatever might happen to my marriage (death or divorce), I just don't believe I could ever fall in love again with a woman or a man. I do not consider the men with whom I have sex as lovers; to me they are sex partners and playmates and that's it. My sex life is not such a calloused syndrome, however, that I have not developed a number of ongoing gay friendships through the years. I guess I could be called a "manizer" just as some men are known as womanizers.

8

Catastrophe Strikes the Gay World and Me Personally

In 1981, a hitherto unknown disease began to decimate the gay population. Early indications were that GRID, as it was called then and later AIDS (Acquired Immune Deficiency Syndrome) was a disease mainly transmitted by homosexual and bisexual men. When scientific research began on Kaposi's sarcoma (a formerly rare cancer which was now increasingly appearing in AIDS patients), the disease was referred to as "gay cancer." As research continued and reports of its progress began appearing in the media, gay communities were literally terrorized by the news. Married bisexual men like myself were having traumas. It appeared that all the hard-fought achievements of the thirty-five-year gay underground and the open gay liberation movement could go down the drain. The organized activists had worked relentlessly to improve the image of the homosexual and now that image was being tarnished more than ever before.

By late 1982, sketchy, inconclusive reports of research from governmental agencies and private organizations had caused hysteria in many circles and was about to create a national crisis.

People thought they could become infected with AIDS by unknowingly using a drinking glass or sitting on a toilet seat that had been used by an infected person. Some dentists and paramedics were wearing, in addition to rubber gloves, protective goggles and screening masks, just in case an infected AIDS victim might breathe on them. Paranoia was running rampant. Then, as AIDS research began to expand on a global scale, more-level heads prevailed.

Eventually, the primary cause of AIDS transmission was found to be anal and vaginal intercourse and the exchanging, consuming, or ingestion of bodily fluids and excrements such as semen, urine, blood, vaginal and penile secretions, and fecal matter. The shared use of unsterile hypodermic needles for injecting intravenous recreational drugs was also targeted as a major route of AIDS infection. Anal intercourse is the favorite sexual practice of many homosexuals and bisexuals. Many times in forceful, vigorous anal intercourse the penetrating partner will tear tissue in the anus and/or rectum of the submissive partner, causing internal bleeding. If the aggressive partner is infected in any way, when he injects his semen, that infection will pass directly into the bloodstream of the submissive partner and may not be discovered until it is much too late. By the same token, if the submissive partner is infected, his infection can travel into the urethra of the aggressive partner. This risk holds true for male and female intercourse, whether vaginal or anal. Likewise, if a gay swallows the semen or excrement of an infected partner, that infection passes into his intestinal tract.

Many homosexuals and bisexuals are at both ends of this situation—they penetrate and are penetrated (aggressive and submissive), often switching roles in the same sexual encounter. In gay parlance, both of these roles are known as Greek (anal intercourse), as opposed to French (oral sex), which may also be either active or passive. Because of the licensed, carte blanche promiscuity of so many gays, all this is the prime source of the havoc caused by AIDS.

Anal intercourse, by far, is the most prevalent means of transmitting the AIDS virus within the gay population. I have never been on the receiving end of anal intercourse. The term "pain in the ass" would certainly apply if I ever let it happen to me. I have one of the tightest ones God ever put in any human. For me, it even hurts to take an enema. It's certainly great, though, that we're not all alike. One time while in one of the baths in San Francisco I was observing a hot and heavy orgy. I heard one of the participants say, "Pull it out, deeper, stud, it hurts so good." For me, pain is not enjoyable. However, for lots of people (male and female), anal intercourse is a pleasurable experience, a fusion of two of the most sensitive organs of two separate bodies, usually culminating in orgasm for one and often times both of the participating parties.

There are many myths about how AIDS is transmitted. First, you can't get it by accident, unless you get stuck by a needle that has gone into an infected person. Think of how very rare such a possibility would be. And everyone should dispell the thought from their minds that you can get AIDS from sitting on a toilet seat! That is impossible unless you're a male sitting on a heap of someone's misguided crap with your penis dangling in it.

In a restaurant, your life is not threatened by a waiter who is infected with AIDS. An infected waiter serving food cannot transmit AIDS. The only way this would be even remotely possible would be if he were to ejaculate into your soup or salad before bringing it to your table—crazy, isn't it? And he absolutely can't pass AIDS on to you by breathing on your food.

Some people think that mosquitoes might transmit AIDS because they draw blood when they bite and fly from one person to another. Scientific study has shown that this is not possible. AIDS is a *sexually* transmitted disease and sex doesn't happen by accident. Eight years of scientific research has concluded that to get AIDS outside of sexual contact is now a long-shot chance in the millions, with the exception of infection through the sharing of unsterile needles.

The hundreds of YMCAs across the country that have fitness and health-club facilities attest to the fact that you can't get AIDS by rubbing elbows with people. As I have stated, the steam rooms and spas are used in the nude. My Y is a very busy and active place. It's not unusual for there to be five, six, or seven men in either the wet or dry steam room at one time. You're sitting in close proximity to one another and breathing in common air. The seating area is almost always wet, indicating that you are sitting in the condensation of sweat from the guy that was there just before you. You may be there in that spot for fifteen or twenty minutes before you go to the showers. If a guy comes in to the same spot, soon after you leave, he'll be sitting in your contribution to the condensation. I doubt very much that anyone has or ever will contract AIDS by using the intimate facilities in a YMCA.

Much about AIDS remains a mystery; how and where the first human contracted the lethal sickness is unknown. However, medical researchers now know that promiscuous behavior encourages the unrestrained transmission and spread of the disease. Innumerable gays throw caution to the wind in selecting sex partners. Indiscriminate promiscuity seems to be the norm in a large portion of the gay population. I suppose one could rationalize by noting that many men seem to be innately uninhibited and gay men even more so. But how could the ravaging AIDS epidemic become a national catastrophe when the carriers of the virus are an ostracized minority of the entire population? Here's an example of how the disease spreads.

Several years ago I was in a popular gay bath in Southern California on a Friday afternoon. The place was alive and jumping with customers. In the center of a large orgy room was an immense round bed. Actually, it was a circular, padded platform raised about a foot above the floor. The room was dimly lighted; nevertheless, you could clearly see what was going on. That pad was vibrating with activity. One particular group caught my eye and I found myself an intense viewer. A very young man, perhaps in his early twenties, was lying naked on his stomach. An older man was on his back penetrating him. It didn't take much imagination to determine when the older guy had his climax. There were a couple of other guys standing nearby waiting their turn. I was anything but naive, just a little astounded. I watched as the other guys took their turns and did their "thing."

In the three hours I was there, I passed through that room four times, stopping to watch five to ten minutes each time. In those three hours, I saw seven different men mounted on and penetrating that young man. It didn't appear that any of the seven had on a condom. Obvious actions indicated that each had an orgasm. If I saw seven, there could have been seven more. I even thought at the time, the semen must have been oozing out of that guy's anus. I didn't particularly enjoy watching, because of the flagrant disregard for health safety. In reality it was a disgusting scene. In view of what has happened in the past seven years, it's inconceivable that this young man could be alive today. He had several sores on his body and it appeared he may have been infected with herpes. He was visibly and outwardly infected with something, but who knew what inwardly. Medical research has established some correlation between certain herpes viruses and that of AIDS. How could decent, intelligent men stoop so low to satisfy their hot and horny sexual cravings?

Anyone or all of those seven men I saw could have been married or had a string of straight girlfriends with whom they had intercourse; these girlfriends, in turn, could have had straight boyfriends with whom they had intercourse, and on and on. Happenings such as this could occur all day long, every day of the year across the country. AIDS is making rapid inroads into the heterosexual population. Could a full-blown national AIDS epidemic become a reality? That reality has been here for some time and AIDS has reached pandemic levels—in its sweep and scope it has transcended epidemc levels. It's spreading like a runaway wildfire out of control.

The promiscuity associated with the spread of AIDS was unwittingly promoted by the gay liberation movement of the 1970s. This movement helped to expand the bathhouse and sex-club business to a $100-million-a-year industry in the United States and Canada. More and more bathhouses were opening and they were becoming ever more popular as a place where gays could find easy sex. I didn't realize it or even believe it at the time, but they were definitely wellsprings of syphilis, gonorrhea, hepatitis, and anal herpes. With promiscuity running rampant, the baths were the prime source of enteric diseases, which are caused by organisms and gastrointestinal parasites in the intestinal tracts of gay men who were continually involved in oral copulation and "rimming." Some medical journals labeled these ailments "gay bowel syndrome." The only limit to promiscuity in the baths was stamina. As a result of the baths, often referred to as "the meat rack," many gay men had 250 or more separate, individual sexual contacts in a year. In the late 1970s and early 1980s, I witnessed lewd, carnal activities in the gay baths on a massive scale, activities that were the harbinger of the coming AIDS catastrophe. It was inevitable that sooner or later there would be a disease outbreak of epidemic proportions in the gay world and now we are living with it in AIDS.

On October 9, 1984, after long political infighting and opposition, Mervyn F. Silverman, M.D., then Public Health Director for the City of San Francisco, using a court order, closed the fourteen gay bathhouses and gay sex clubs in the city. I had many ecstatic sexual experiences in a number of those commercial establishments and was somewhat nostalgic on learning of their closure, even though I now fully realized the baths were literally biological cesspools of infection. God has been good to me and my wife. Only once in all my promiscuous double life have I brought home an infection (clap) and I thank Him that she didn't get it.

When I traveled extensively around the country for the XYZ Group, I came to the realization there could be at least two hundred and perhaps as many as three hundred gay bathhouses from coast to coast. I've been gone from the gay bath scene for more than seven years; it's been that long since I've been in one. The gay baths today, where they still exist, are spawning grounds for AIDS. Those who still patronize them have absolutely no regard for their own health safety and that of others. Safe sex is a thing of the past, unless in a monogamous relationship and this is paramount when it comes to the gay world. I read newspaper accounts from time to time about gay baths being closed in various places by new city ordinances and health department mandates. In view of the dreadful AIDS publicity, I don't see how any remain in business. Even if an AIDS vaccine were developed and marketed, and the baths should become popular again, I doubt very much that I would return to the gay bath scene.

The following is a quote from a report on the AIDS epidemic in the January 12, 1987 issue of *U.S. News & World Report*:

> The Centers for Disease Control estimates that 1.5 million Americans now carry the virus but display no symptoms. Others think that number may be as high as 4 million. Conceivably, all these people could progress to the incurable disease, certainly a fourth to a half will. With no effective cure in sight, all those who fall sick are doomed. . . . So far, AIDS has killed an estimated total of 1,370 heterosexuals. The toll will pass 15,000 by 1991.

And that is heterosexuals—think of how staggering the number is for homosexuals. *U.S. News & World Report* stated, "Up to 10 million people worldwide now carry the AIDS virus and are potential victims."

The depressing media coverage of the AIDS crisis was getting to me. I began thinking of my gay promiscuity; in the time frame of 1981–82 when AIDS was just coming into the limelight. Even though I was reasonably sure I was not a carrier of the AIDS virus, there is a significant difference between being reasonably sure and positively sure. It became a gnawing contemplation. For one thing, I had been a recent blood donor. Then, too, I had my wife to think about and it was weighing heavy on my mind. Finally, in early March 1987, I bit the bullet and secretly went for the HTLV-III Antibody Test. This was the blood test, at that time, that showed whether or not you're a carrier of the AIDS virus. Now, it's the HIV Antibody Test.

In most places, the AIDS test is done on a highly confidential basis, at no cost, through the county health department. When I gave my first blood sample, I was given a small receipt with a twice-verified identification number and was told that the test result would be available in two weeks. The blood sample went to a state-controlled AIDS testing laboratory. The procedure assures that there will be no violation of anyone's identity. I was strictly a number.

And now, the punch line: I do *not* have AIDS and I'm *not* a carrier of the AIDS virus. It cost me absolutely nothing and I have returned twice since then and had it redone, just to reassure my peace of mind. Evidently, I was not as promiscuous as I thought I had been. Perhaps I was a little more selective in choosing my sex partners than were Rock Hudson and Liberace. On the other hand, God may have extended just a little more good luck in my direction. He knows my family is proud of me and they need me. It was, indeed, reassuring to know that in the two-year period prior to my first AIDS test the blood I gave on two separate occasions to the American Red Cross, for a humanitarian cause, was not contaminated.

With the deaths of Rock Hudson in October 1985 and Liberace in February 1987, a new focus was placed on the sobering and grim consequences of the AIDS catastrophe. Hudson was an avowed homosexual and undoubtedly proud of it, while Liberace never wanted the world to know he was homosexual. Hudson admitted he had AIDS and by doing so became somewhat of a courageous hero in the ongoing battle to eradicate the incurable killer disease. It seemed almost inevitable that Rock Hudson, the most notable gay actor in Hollywood, would be the first of the superstars to knowingly die from AIDS.

Liberace, on the other hand, had hoped to keep the world from knowing he died from AIDS; he was a man of inordinate pride. It's strange that Liberace had such an intense propensity for concealing his homosexuality when, in fact, his very demeanor and lifestyle were the epitome of flamboyant homosexuality. It appeared that there was almost a covert cover-up by Liberace's confidants and physician to hide the cause of his death, even to the extent that their actions provoked a public confrontation with the county coroner. There was a marked similarity in the appearance and emaciated condition of the bodies of the two celebrities (Rock Hudson and Liberace) in the weeks just prior to their deaths. The deaths of these two notables let the world know that homosexuality is for real and AIDS is a ravaging, fatal by-product. Before this AIDS thing is over, the world will surely know there are a hell of a lot of homosexuals among us.

A short time ago this tragic, ongoing AIDS disaster struck home. My wife and I learned that a dear, young, longtime family friend was stricken with the disease and was given only six months to live. When we found out about this tragedy, Eric had already started losing weight, so it seemed likely that he would waste away in the predicted period of time. Eric was only thirty-four years old, and although he was a confirmed bachelor, even I had never suspected him of being gay. He was a young executive, headed straight up the corporate ladder. When we learned of the sad news, Sue was dumbfounded and in a state of shock for several days. She said to me, "I can't believe Eric is gay. You just never know about people, do you? Even the ones you're so close to." I said, "Yes honey, you never know."

Only four and a half months later, Eric died from viral pneumonia brought on by AIDS. His parents, lifelong friends of Sue and me, have been totally crushed ever since. However, they had some time to prepare for this. When they learned their son had only six months to live, they invited him back home to live out his last days. AIDS was merciless to Eric; it didn't even give him the six months the doctors predicted.

The world is beginning to know that AIDS is the leprosy of the twentieth century and it's all around us. This lethal disease was unheard of by most people eight years ago. Today it's on everyone's mind and it's now an inescapable reality.

The plight of the AIDS victims has captured the hearts of millions of Americans. Innumerable physicians, scientists, and others involved in AIDS research are homosexual and have a very personal stake in the outcome. A number of these individuals have died from the dreaded disease. It appears now that before a cure or a vaccine is found, billions of dollars will be spent in combating AIDS. The 1987 edition of the *Encyclopedia of Associations* lists twenty-one AIDS-related organizations. They consist of governmental and congressional lobbyists in pursuit of the astronomical funds needed for AIDS research. They are also made up of information, education, and service groups involving epidemiologists, physicians, medical scientists, clinical researchers, and AIDS victims themselves.

Numerous illustrious celebrities are giving their time and

talents to soliciting funds for AIDS research. Even though AIDS is primarily a gay man's disease, many women seem to have a special compassion for the cause. As early as June 1983, a fund-raiser was hosted by actress Debbie Reynolds in San Francisco for the KS/AIDS Foundation. Shirley MacLaine appeared in the same show. For a number of years Elizabeth Taylor has been the Founding National Chairperson of the American Foundation for AIDS Research (AmFAR). Dr. Mervyn Silverman, former head of the San Francisco Department of Public Health, is president of AmFAR which has offices in New York City and Los Angeles. A few of the notable names that appear on the AmFAR National Council roster include Barbra Streisand, Woody Allen, Mrs. Lyndon Baines Johnson, Douglas Fairbanks, Jr., Rosalyn Carter, Tony Randall, Raquel Welch, Warren Beatty, Angela Lansbury, Burt Bacharach, and Phil Donahue. Prior to his death, the name of Leonard Bernstein appeared.

Even though Elizabeth Taylor is a classic prototype of feminine pulchritude, and in spite of her many marriages, she has long displayed an affinity for and magnetism toward gay men. In addition to her relationship with Malcolm Forbes, she had a close and lengthy relationship with Rock Hudson. Since the onset of the AIDS crisis, Miss Taylor has given a great abundance of her time and resources to the groundswell for eradication of the deadly disease. She is dedicated to the AIDS cause.

The shocking announcement by basketball superstar Earvin "Magic" Johnson in November 1991 that he has the AIDS virus had an astounding impact on millions of adults and kids who viewed him as an idol; I hope they still do. He is a fine human being. At the time of the announcement, Johnson didn't admit or deny that he is gay, but if so, he is bisexual. Two months before he learned that he has the virus, he married his college sweetheart. We could give him the benefit of the doubt. A small percentage of all AIDS is now being transmitted between heterosexuals. Johnson's new wife tested negative.

"Magic" Johnson is only one in a six-year succession of American celebrities who have tested positive for the HIV virus. He has been given a death sentence, just like the others, unless an arresting drug is discovered in the very near future. Another notable personality, who like Rock Hudson and Liberace died from AIDS, was Roy Cohn, the famous gay New York lawyer; he died from AIDS in August 1986. Cohn was a personal friend and counselor to both church cardinals and crime mobsters. At one time, he was chief counsel for U.S. Senator Joseph McCarthy, the controversial communist-hunter.

The world may never know the true impact of the AIDS tragedy. I have personal suspicions that a number of VIP personalities have died or are dying from AIDS. I predict that in the future the world will be jolted by the disclosure of the AIDS deaths of some of our most prominent and renowned personalities, people with the guts of Rock Hudson who thought the world should know. Having a promiscuous sex life in this day and age is like playing Russian roulette, and still there are millions of people who keep playing the deadly game.

The AIDS crisis is actually encouraging promiscuous sexuality, both hetero and homo, among the youth of our nation. Many universities and now high schools, without pretense or restraint, are making free condoms available to students. Some have even installed condom vending machines in conspicuous locations throughout the campus. This is true of most of the University of California campuses, including Berkeley and UCLA, and also most of the campuses of the California State University System. According to the American College Health Association in Rockville, Maryland, free condoms on campus are becoming widespread across the country. Avoiding AIDS has become a routine procedure on the campuses of numerous universities and colleges. And now certain government agencies and private organizations are dispensing quantities of free, disposable, sterile, hypodermic needles to recreational drug users in a desperate effort to control the spread of AIDS among intra-venous drug addicts.

In the great offensive against AIDS, free condoms are also being dispensed to the inmate population in most men's prisons in this country. Anal intercourse runs rampant and unchecked in the cells, exercise yards, and various surreptitious areas of these institutions. Correctional officers checking beds at night turn their heads the other way and ignore it; in most places they have been instructed to do so. Sodomy has always been a way of life for an untold number of those confined in penal institutions.

Now researchers believe a million and a half Americans are carriers of the AIDS virus; some even believe the figure could be closer to three million. By the end of 1991, full-blown AIDS had struck 206,843 Americans, killing 133,232 of them. Those who have it know an early, impending death is their destiny. By mid-June 1988, one American was stricken with AIDS every fourteen minutes, according to the Centers for Disease Control. That is equivalent to approximately 102 new AIDS cases every day in the United States or 102 new imminent deaths, and the statistics are climbing. AIDS has now taken the lives of many more Americans than the 58,000 who died in combat in the eight-year Vietnam War.

One of my passions, in the writing of this book, was to give the whole world a frank, uninhibited, realistic scrutiny and overview of AIDS, the most disastrous and tragic health crisis of this century. I believe my candid narration here gives a far greater comprehension of the killer disease than the brochure of former Surgeon General C. Everett Koop, "Understanding AIDS." I'm sure the good doctor's staff had a difficult time in coping with propriety when drafting copy for the mailer that went into every mailbox across the land in the second quarter of 1988. When there's such an urgent message to be told, you shouldn't "pussyfoot" around about it. The message truly was urgent. This terrifying disease has no compassion or mercy for anyone in its course of destruction. It should make everyone shudder when they think of who might be next—a friend, a loved one; it could be anyone.

I thank God I don't have AIDS, but I have been plagued with another curse as the result of my bisexuality. Even though it's not imminently life-threatening, it has made my life hell, off and on, for the past ten years. About seventeen years ago my friend Sandy, the owner of the beauty salon in Berkeley, introduced me to a new "kick." It is a chemical substance used by the medical profession in the treatment of angina pectoris, a painful symptom of heart disease. The substance is amyl nitrate, a liquid inhalant that opens the blood vessels for a rush of blood and oxygen to the brain. A couple of whiffs cause an erotic sensation in the sensitive nerve areas of the tongue, penis, and anus. In some cases it prolongs orgasm and may relax the sphincter muscle, making anal intercourse more enjoyable for those who find it painful. In those days, Sandy got the real thing from a pharmacist friend. Legally it was available only on prescription. The product is produced by a pharmaceutical manufacturer in the form of small gauze-wrapped ampules that can be broken with the squeeze of the fingers, much like spirits-of-ammonia ampules.

Amyl nitrate added an indescribable thrill and excitement to gay sex. After three or four times, I believe I became obsessively addicted to the stuff. It was about this time that black-market entrepreneurs were getting into the act. If they couldn't get the ingredients to produce nitrate, they would produce nitrite which has the same sensual effect. You could buy it, under the counter, in little unmarked brown bottles that would contain about two thimbles full. It was a clear liquid acid and its effectiveness would last about a month, depending on how many times the cap had been removed. You could buy it in most gay bars, adult bookstores, and gay baths. The product in its tiny brown bottle became known as "poppers." For years it was the prime aphrodisiac of the gay world.

About twelve to fifteen years ago, a number of the black-market producers turned legitimate and began manufacturing their product with the blessing of the various government agencies having jurisdiction over such an enterprise. There were numerous brands sold openly on the market, attractively packaged in the same little brown bottles, but with captivating professional labels. They were on sale almost everywhere in gay businesses. Most of these substitute products were either butyl or alkyl nitrites or nitrates. They had very much the same effect as the medical amyl nitrate. Amyl was the champagne and butyl and alkyl were the beer of the "popper" orbit. Depending on the product and where purchased, "poppers" usually sold for $4.50 to $7.00 in the gay establishments.

For several years I wouldn't engage in gay sex without sniffing the liquid acid. Then, about twelve years ago a strange malady entered my life. It lasted only two weeks, but it was two weeks of torment and hell. I had agonizing pains in my head that would come and go. About the time I decided I couldn't take it any longer and had to see a doctor, the pains disappeared.

Two years later the head pains recurred with much greater intensity and lasted about a month. After a couple of weeks, I decided to go to the family physician. He had a simple cranial X-ray taken as well as some lab tests and was about to send me to a neurologist. Then, the pains disappeared just as they had two years before. During that month I refrained from using nitrite, although I did not seriously think of it then as being the cause of my problem. However, I capitulated and began using the acid inhalant just as frequently again.

Some months later the head pains returned with a vengeance. This time I really was in trouble. The pains were so relentless and excruciating I couldn't function. It was impossible to work and if I needed to go somewhere, my wife or one of my associates or employees would have to drive me. The pains were like detonating shock waves—electric current going through my head and brain. If I was talking on the telephone and a jolt hit, I might drop the phone. For a few seconds I couldn't talk and for an hour or so I could be totally disoriented.

My family physician referred me to a neurologist, who had me examined by an oncologist and a radiologist. I had an extensive series of X-rays taken, including a brain CAT scan, numerous lab tests, and ultimately an MRI brain scan. All this dispelled the possibility of a tumor or cancer. After consultation, the three doctors diagnosed my condition as tic douloureux. Through a sequence of events, I was referred to a renowned university neurosurgeon, and after reviewing all the reports and X-rays, the expert said the diagnosis was irrelevant. He said the main thing is the cause, not the condition. He informed me that a blood vessel or artery in my head had expanded and was touching the trigeminal nerve. When the contact becomes unrestrained, the pressure triggers an impulse that causes the tics or shock waves, producing torturous pain along with such side reactions as mental confusion. He said the prognosis was that I would survive with this disorder, but the only way to eradicate it from my life once and for all was through cerebrovascular/microneurosurgery. The procedure sets apart the expanded blood vessel from the trigeminal nerve. In the meantime, he prescribed a medication that brought the pain under control. The condition lasted five months, and it was during that time that through my absurd, irrational conduct and execution in business negotiations, I was forced into Chapter XI Bankruptcy. Eventually, as I stated before, my wife and I were wiped out financially.

While writing this book, I have had another attack of tic douloureux/trigeminal neuralgia, and it has been ongoing for some time. The medication is working, although it produces risky, negative side effects. While taking the drug, I have to have monthly blood tests to keep the side effects under surveillance.

At one time, a slight overdose put me in a state of violent convulsions and I thought I would surely die. The operation may be inevitable.

In the past five years, when these torturous seizures have hit, Sue will become so anguished that it almost appears she feels my pain. Her compassion has sustained me many times. She assures me that God is only letting this happen so I may attain a higher place in heaven. I could never let her know that this curse was brought on by my sexual lust and deviation. Whether or not my continual sniffing of the acid did any damage to my lungs, I do not know. However, I have had bronchial pneumonia twice in the past two years and never before. Was it worth it? If I only knew when I got started on the stuff what I know now, this would never have happened.

I didn't believe "poppers" could be a dangerous health hazard because the drug was allowed by the Federal Food and Drug Administration to be sold openly as a sexual stimulant. When I traveled extensively for the XYZ Group, I saw the acid chemicals for sale openly in such places as Dallas, New Orleans, Kansas City, Washington, D.C., Boston, Chicago, New York's Times Square, and San Francisco's Tenderloin. In some of the gay bars, gay baths, adult bookstores, and gay motels, the product was promoted and merchandised with point-of-purchase advertising posters furnished by the various name-brand manufacturers. Some of the brand names were Locker Room, Aroma of Man, Rush, Blackjack, Wildcat, Bolt, Heart On, Quicksilver, and Bullet, to name just a few. The advertising was very professional and effective.

Very early on in AIDS research, and its relation to Kaposi's sarcoma, "poppers" were considered as a possible source or contributing factor. However, that theory was soon abandoned. It was estimated that in 1980 alone, some five million doses of nitrate inhalants were purchased by gays in America. The manufacture and sale of "poppers" was big business. Nevertheless, some local jurisdictions in the mid-1980s were beginning to ban public sale of these acid products. In Los Angeles County, an ordinance banning the sale of the chemicals went into effect in November 1986. The new law was immediately challenged in a court suit by one of the manufacturers of the product. On December 19, 1986, an article appeared in the *Los Angeles Times* with the heading "Judge Backs County Ban on Poppers." The day before a superior court judge upheld and refused to throw out the new county ordinance banning the public sale of the aphrodisiac chemical. Finally, in February 1991, a federal law went into effect making the sale of "poppers" illegal in the United States.

In the years that I had used these acid inhalants, they gave me an ecstatic, delirious high in my gay sexual encounters. However, there was a latent effect that caused the negatives of using the drug to outweigh the positives. The brain surgeon described the pain of tic douloureaux as being perhaps the most excruciating, torturous pain known to humans. I finally came to the realization that my habitual use of the acid inhalant was the cause of the malady that was ruining my life. The prescribed medical therapeutic use of amyl nitrate is for opening blood vessels. Now there is little doubt in my mind that my addiction to and the continuous snorting of the acid, for seventeen years, has permanently enlarged a blood vessel that touches a major sensory nerve in my head. I haven't used "poppers" in some time and as I'm getting older, gay sex seems to have as much allure and enjoyment as it did when I was sniffing the stuff. I may still have to have the brain surgery, but I'm hoping with a little help from God, this too shall pass.

We live only once. If we pass through this world without having experienced a little of everything, we will never know what we missed. I should, however, qualify this statement by saying that most of us ought to live life to the fullest, but not get hooked on something that will shorten our lives mentally and physically. We all have it within our power to determine whether we will let drugs, liquor, or the threat of AIDS have a ruinous effect on our lives. The astute adventurer proceeds with extreme caution. Obviously, I was neither astute nor cautious in my use of "poppers."

9

God and Religion—
The Homosexual Dilemma

Faith and Sexuality

I have frequently made reference to God throughout this book. You may be wondering what this lecherous guy with all these erotic activities in his life knows about God. It may surprise you to know that God and I have become very close friends in the past ten years. Prior to that, He was a thorn in my side and made my life miserable. Then, there was a big change in my attitudes. The point is, God didn't change; I changed.

I finally came to the realization that God is not my enemy, but my very best and closest friend. It's really sad that thirty years went by before I comprehended this, yet it took that long to adjust my religious mores. God didn't create the mores; we human beings have made the mores and what we have created we can change. After I made some changes in my mores, I liberated myself from the syndrome of agonizing guilt, and today I have a much better perception of God and know that He understands me. I am now thoroughly convinced that He is not going to condemn me to everlasting damnation in the fires of hell for my sexual preferences and enjoyment here on earth. My soul is a spiritual being, but if it did go to Satan's inferno, it would become spiritual ashes in a short time and it would be all over anyway.

There are some holier-than-thou moralist Christians who would condemn me and my lifestyle. They think that God sent the ravaging disease AIDS as a warning to our permissive society. I might have fallen for this explanation ten years ago, but not today. One of the greatest lies the devil has successfully perpetrated down through the ages is that an angry God sends us sickness, misfortune, suffering, and death in order to teach us a lesson. This despicable lie is believed and accepted by millions upon millions of Christians today. The devil has a vested interest in seeing to it that we view God from a position of trembling fear. He wants us to believe that if we do not choose God's way, God will retaliate with all these calamities. The devil knows if we really believe this, we will ultimately reject God outright. Such a picture of God is utterly ludicrous. God is love and compassion and the source of all good. God did not send us AIDS.

Before I had worked all this out in my mind, my guilt complex was destroying my life. When I finally got over my self-pity, I came to the conclusion that there are two categories of people, gay and non-gay, and perhaps I was fortunate being some of both in spite of the psychological quandary it was causing in my life.

I suppose using the term "non-gay" is a throwback to my Catholic upbringing. I was born and raised a Catholic and will probably always be a Catholic of sorts. When I was growing up, you were either Catholic or non-Catholic. That was in the days when the church was bent on global conquest. The church's objective was to bring into the fold hundreds of millions of souls from every region of this earth. It was a conquest very much like that of its arch enemy, Communism, in the past half century.

When Pope John XXIII arrived on the scene in 1958, the church took a new direction. He was the instigator of Vatican II, the Second Ecumenical Council, which opened in October 1962. It was the start of an overwhelming reformation within the church. One of its objectives was to make the church more understanding toward the non-Catholic world. Another objective was to make the basic doctrine of the church more acceptable and tolerable to the multitude of the faithful and to make the liturgy understandable to the laity. In the latter regard, the Mass was changed from Latin to the vernacular language of each country where Catholicism is practiced (English in the United States). There were numerous changes in the precepts of the church. Catholics could now marry non-Catholics and Catholics could become Freemasons. But the change that blew my mind was allowing Catholics to eat meat on Friday. When I was a child and even a young adult, I believed one of the most serious sins I could commit was to eat meat on Friday. I was taught that if I did it intentionally and were to die before I could get to confession and repent for that sin, I was doomed to purgatory or limbo. Today, in the church, there is no such thing as limbo; it was done away with in Vatican II. It was a figment of man's imagination, as is much of the dogma of the church. So, I have adjusted my mores, just as the church has adjusted its doctrine, and life is now so much more worth living.

With his death in June 1963, Pope John XXIII had a short reign. He was considered by many of the old-line thinkers in the church to be a zealous rabble-rouser. They are probably the ones who believe reform should take a gradual course, not come about rapidly, but evolve over a period of a hundred or a hundred and fifty years.

Despite my disagreement with certain tenets of Catholic dogma, I would be the first to admit that religion has played a prodigious role in the development of a structured society, which is the basis of our orderly civilization. In my opinion, if it were not for religion, we would all be human animals sniffing each other's genitals out in the middle of the street and having sex with our parents and children. Nevertheless, I believe the Roman Catholic Church has gone too far in its strategy of instilling a guilt complex in everyone. For centuries, the confessional has been the means of keeping the flock on the straight and narrow path. If a sinner has to repent for his sins, he will be reluctant to perpetuate moral offenses. Yet even in this area, the church is softening its stance. Confession is no longer called confession—it is now known as "reconciliation." Webster's defines reconcile as settle, resolve, and adapt. There are two sides in every reconciliation and each must adapt. My interpretation is that the church is attempting to adapt. Still today, at holy communion in the Mass, the words are said, "Lord I am not worthy to receive you. Only say the word and my soul shall be healed." If a homosexual believes everything he has ever read in the Bible, he must also believe that his soul shall not be healed. I know now that God is not scornful. The Bible is a book of interpretation—what is right for me may be wrong for you, and what is right for you may be wrong for me. Even a clock that has long been stopped is right twice a day.

I just can't believe that, because I have had sex with both women and men in this life, it will have a bearing on where I go in the hereafter. I can't quite understand heaven, anyway, as it is sometimes depicted by theologians. It sounds to me like the dullest place out of this world—a place where I wouldn't want to be caught dead. But, if there is a next world, I believe gays, like other mortals of this world, will have positions of honor in heaven. Our time is so limited on planet earth there is no reason why we shouldn't enjoy it to the fullest and still honor the God that put us here.

Catholic Doctrine vs. the Gay Believer

John XXIII left many issues unresolved, perhaps the most grave and crucial of which is homosexuality—not just in the laity, but also within the clergy. This is an issue the church would like to sweep under the rug. Nonetheless, it can't continue much longer to keep its head buried in the sand in regard to this humanitarian issue. I have often thought that I could test the church's policy on bisexuality by applying to the proper tribunal in Rome for a dispensation for my bisexual status. On the other hand, I might get excommunicated.

The subject of homosexuality shouldn't be such a mind-boggling matter. It's been around for thousands of years and the church has been dealing with it for centuries. In the Holy Bible homosexual acts are described as "sodomy," a word that, until the past twenty or twenty-five years, had a vile connotation. Today, we more commonly refer to this kind of fulfilling, gratifying sex as anal intercourse and oral copulation. And, of course, these sexual acts are commonly practiced by numerous heterosexual couples. Some practice them to circumvent pregnancy and abortion. I suppose you might call it a natural form of contraception. Reputable psychiatrists and marriage counselors recommend these diversions to certain heterosexual couples whose sex desires are waning or perhaps totally dissipated. These sex acts are part of the come-back therapy. In many people they create a new excitement and an awakening, which some psychologists say have saved many marriages from hitting the rocks.

I strongly feel that the Catholic Church should follow the lead of many protestant churches, which recognize gays as righteous, honorable people and have special services and functions for them. Not so with the Catholic Church. How much longer can the church ignore this catastrophic dilemma? A serious and significant rift has developed within the church regarding homo-

sexuality. It involves hinterland and metropolitan clergy, theologians, and the hierarchy. Many compassionate bishops, archbishops, and certain theologians are expressing their benevolent
and sympathetic views toward homosexuals and bisexuals. Other
theologians contend that the extensive, universal spread of homosexuality would threaten the very existence of the human race
and bring about its eventual extinction, and that the integrity and
decency of the family home and social structure could not be
maintained if homosexual activity was not condemned by moral
codes and public opinion, and made punishable by governmental law. Such reasoning ignores the fact that the existent human
species has managed to survive in spite of its widespread homosexual activity through the centuries. Sexual relations between
men seem to be extensive in certain cultures such as Moslem
and Buddhist, which are more seriously concerned with problems
of overpopulation than they are with any threat of underpopula-
tion. Strangely enough, these are also cultures in which the institution of the family is very strong. This extinction theory doesn't
hold water. Homosexuality is not going to do away with God,
motherhood, and the American flag. I'm gay and at the same
time a good husband and loving father, and of recent years a
respected and venerated grandfather.

Could it be that a continuing defection from the ranks of
the clergy is stirring a change of attitude in the church? Undoubtedly many of these departures are the outgrowth of celibacy. The confined communal environment of many rectories,
convents, abbeys, and monasteries, where men are living with
men and women with women, must put a severe strain on the
vows of chastity and arouse inclinations of homosexuality—after
all, they are only human.

A small segment of the hierarchy has begun to take church
doctrine into its own hands in a desperate effort to cope with
the reality of homosexuality. However, they are being censured
by the Vatican and castigated by the universal church. A prime

example is Archbishop Raymond Hunthausen of the Seattle, Washington archdiocese. For a number of years, Hunthausen had openly expressed his compassion and sympathy for individuals affected by church restraint in areas of family life and personal behavior, principally homosexuality. Finally, in 1986 the Holy See stripped Hunthausen of all authority. Papal power versus the new wave of collegial decision making by United States bishops became a source of painful contention for the Supreme Pontiff. Three high-ranking American prelates took up the Hunthausen cause through the powerful political process within the church. Early in 1987 Hunthausen's authority was restored. It was done in such a way that the Vatican could save face and it appeared that Rome had not backed down. Neverthless, it let the whole world know that the Vatican and the American Catholic Church is struggling with the matter of homosexuality. The Roman Catholic Church is a centuries-old, inherently conservative institution which takes centuries to ingest all aspects of uncommon, unconventional human behavior. However, the day of the homosexual is upon us and the church knows it without a doubt.

Many American bishops, archbishops, and theologians are bending an ear to an organization called "Dignity." Dignity is a composition of Catholic gays and lesbians and includes in its membership many prominent church-supporting individuals. Perhaps the voice of Dignity will eventually make such a resounding echo that it will be heard in Rome.

In late 1989 another scandal rocked the church. It was revealed that Father Bruce Ritter, the sixty-three-year-old Franciscan priest who founded Covenant House in New York City, was sexually involved with a number of his male charges. Ritter started the shelter twenty years before in humble circumstances for teenage runaway drug addicts, prostitutes, alcoholics, and those seeking refuge from the brutality of child abuse. The institution grew to an $85 million budget with a paid staff of

1,700 and about 2,000 volunteer workers in seventeen shelters in the U.S., Canada, Mexico, Guatemala, Honduras, and Panama. In 1984, President Reagan called Ritter an "unsung hero" in his State of the Union address. President George Bush visited the Covenant House center at Times Square in New York City in June of 1989 and referred to Ritter as one of the brightest of the nation's "thousand points of light." The revelation did more than tarnish Father Ritter's sterling reputation as a compassionate benefactor of youth; he was forced to resign as president of Covenant House.

A more recent embarrassment for the church was the much publicized sexual escapades of fifty-six-year-old Archbishop Eugene Marino of the Atlanta, Georgia Archdiocese. It was disclosed in the media in August 1990 that Marino had an ongoing sexual relationship with twenty-seven-year-old Vicki Long, a lay minister of the archdiocese. Marino now is in church-imposed seclusion in an unrevealed location.

The church is made up of men and as long as there are men, there will be conflicts of morality. Who is to say what is moral and what is immoral when it comes to an individual's human rights? Man makes the laws, rules, and regulations and if it's legally permissible, it should be morally acceptable. Many of my perceptions about gay life and Christianity are corroborated in two books by Father John J. McNeill, S.J.—*The Church and The Homosexual* and *Taking a Chance on God*. McNeill, himself an admitted homosexual, psychotherapist, and moral theologian, was expelled from his order in the fall of 1987 for articulating perspectives that could radically alter traditional sexual ethics and conduct. When more than 50,000 copies of the first edition of his first book were in print, the Catholic Church banned all of Father McNeill's work. The Jesuit order produces more intellectual scholars than any other ecclesiastic entity in the church and many are involved in research outside of pure theology. When some are bold enough to tell it as it is, they are castigated as rabble-rousing demagogues.

The Bible was written by men of childlike intellects and suppositions (by today's standards), who believed the world was flat. They couldn't comprehend that a man would ever go to the moon, and to discuss any concept outside their simple notions was heresy. Today, in the twentieth century, we are beneficiaries of scientific enlightenment and in many ways are intellectually superior to our ancient ancestors. Perhaps we know something the wise men of old and drafters of the Bible didn't know. One thing we certainly know is that homosexuality is as real as the people involved and to thwart it would mean the ruination of millions and millions of lives.

I firmly believe the time has come to face up to and challenge the hypocrisy within the church regarding homosexual priests. They like other priests consecrate and lay hands on the Body and Blood of Christ and distribute it to the faithful.

The Celibate Clergy—How Long?

Celibacy has always been a consequential problem among the clergy in the church. However, it was usually heterosexual problems that would come to light. The mythical Ralph Cardinal de Bricassart in *The Thorn Birds* is a preeminent example. Undoubtedly, there are many Father Ralphs today. Not so mythical were the extracurricular activities of a certain American cardinal a short time ago. John Patrick Cardinal Cody, archbishop of Chicago, the nation's largest Roman Catholic archdiocese, created an agonizing, disgraceful embarrassment for the church. Cody was a powerful ecclesiastical figure who enjoyed strong papal support throughout his fifty years in the priesthood, including his years as archbishop of New Orleans, all this in spite of his oppposition to certain reforms adopted during the Second Vatican Council. His authoritarian administration of his archdiocese erupted in scandal in late 1981. Insiders accused His Eminence of diverting a million dollars in church funds to a longtime single lady "friend" to keep her in a style of luxury. The disclosure of the allegations prompted a federal grand jury investigation. For him, it was a diversion of funds; for me, it would have been embezzlement. Sensational stories and articles on the scandal appeared in the *Chicago Tribune* in September 1981. Follow-up coverage appeared again in the *Tribune* in October, November, and December of that same year. Cody's death at the height of the scandal, in April 1982, was very timely. Even though this prince of the church was caught with his hands in the cookie jar, it's hard to believe his soul is in hell for all eternity. Who knows what he gave up for Lent; it may have bought him time. Cody was seventy-four when he died; sounds like he was a pretty good man after all. I only hope I will be as virile at seventy-four.

The celibacy rule of the church is now confronted with one of its most serious challenges in modern history—that of homosexuality among the clergy. There are gay priests actively engaged in homosexuality. This headline appeared on the front page of the *San Francisco Examiner,* Sunday, January 4, 1987: "AIDS Among the Clergy—A Public Test of Faith." The opening sentence in the article read, "AIDS has spread into the Catholic priesthood and stricken at least a dozen clergy, according to interviews with Catholic clergy and church leaders across the nation." The article referred to the church's iron-door secrecy on the matter, but indicated an unknown number of priests have died from AIDS. The article candidly referred to a San Francisco priest stricken with and dying from AIDS. The pigeons have come home to roost.

Since AIDS is primarily a sexually transmitted disease, its presence among men publicly committed to celibacy, through vows of chastity, raises grave questions about hypocrisy within the church. If a member of the hierarchy were to die from

AIDS, surely such a scandalous disclosure would never reach the press; he would probably die in a Catholic hospital. Homosexuality is not a problem confined to just the clergy of the Catholic Church. Most of the major Protestant denominations including Episcopal, Presbyterian, Lutheran, and Methodist are confronted with the same problem. However, they have one thing in their favor—they're not grappling with the implications of celibacy.

There are a number of reasons why celibacy has become a festering frustration within the clergy of the church. In the United States today there are more than fifty married priests with families. For the most part, they are defectors from the Episcopal church where marriage and family life is normal for priests. They have been reordained in the Catholic church, causing great consternation among many of the 53,000 American priests bound by their celibate vow of chastity. Furthermore, in the first few hundred years in the history of the church, there were more than forty married popes. A few years ago a confidential survey of priests in this country concluded that 65 percent of U.S. priests would prefer non-celibacy. A similar survey showed that 72 percent of American Catholics believe their priests should have the right to marry.

Constrained celibacy causes moral conflicts with some members of the clergy. On the "Larry King Live Show" on national network television (September 14, 1990), King had as his guest a former Jesuit priest. Father Terrance Sweeney, S.J., had been suspended by his order, the Society of Jesus, and ultimately stripped of his ecclesiastical authority by Rome for his research on celibacy. Sweeney said that in past years United States bishops and other church authorities have paid more than $100,000,000 in coverup money for priests involved in sexually exploiting children, both girls and boys.

Even though priests are expected to be the epitome of virtue, some feel they are entitled to just one unobtrusive vice.

Since they haven't taken vows to abstain from all good things in life, that one vice for some is partaking of spirits, and not holy spirits. From time to time bishops send subordinate priests to substance-abuse centers for alcoholic-treatment programs. When I think of all the revealed hypocrisy within the church, it relieves my conscience.

Birth Control, Abortion, and the Population Time Bomb

The church must change its attitude in many areas, but especially in regard to birth control. The church is fostering a tragic, ruinous, worldwide humanitarian, ecological, and economic catastrophe, all stemming from overpopulation, which is overburdening our natural resources. Within a small segment of clergy in the church, there is a shrouded split over contraception and pro-life vs. pro-choice. Some even view it as a partisan political or social issue rather than a moral issue. In fact, despite the church's diametric opposition to abortion, numerous priests and even members of the hierarchy were against the confirmation of Clarence Thomas as an associate justice of the Supreme Court regardless of his pro-life stance. It shouldn't be a startling revelation—after all, there are more than 53,000 Catholic priests in the United States, many involved in liberal politics. I personally believe abortion is murder; however, there are men of the cloth who are not convinced. Moreover, I believe contraception is a humane alternative to abortion and the church must face the reality that it can't have it both ways—no birth control and no abortion.

When one looks at all of the issues confronting Catholic dogma today—homosexuality, clerical celibacy, birth control, abortion, divorce, use of condoms in AIDS prevention, etc.—it is obvious that sex is the blockbuster issue facing the church now and in the immediate future.

Scandals in Protestant Churches

The problems of sexuality and the corruption of the clergy are not confined to the Catholic Church. Shocking scandals have also tainted the reputations of various Protestant denominations. You may recall in the mid 1970s the Reverend Jim Jones, a prominent Protestant clergyman in California, took more than 900 of his followers to South America to establish a religious commune in a jungle in Guyana. Weird stories began to come back to relatives in this country from the Jones followers depicting the sinister life in the commune. In November 1978 a United States congressman and four members of his party, investigating conditions at the commune, were ambushed and killed. When Jones faced the reality that his ulterior motives were about to be revealed, he led his devotees in a mass suicide and was responsible for nearly 900 deaths, including his own. Jones had acquired millions of dollars in assets from his followers and was sexually involved with members of his cult.

In early 1987, the dynasty of television evangelism was rocked by corruption—sex scandals and misappropriation of funds, involving millions of dollars. No doubt, the famous TV evangelists believe in God, but some get caught up in earthly situations, things they wouldn't want their millions of viewers to be involved in. Their "holy war" erupted into a sanctimonious circus with Jim Bakker of the PTL Club as the deposed ring master. The little scamp that blew the whistle and revealed Bakker's lust for worldly gratification, as you may recall, is one Jessica Hahn. She said she was a virgin when she met Jim Bakker that December afternoon in 1980 in a Tampa, Florida, beach hotel room. According to Hahn, when Bakker and his associate Rev. John Wesley Fletcher were finished with her, she was ravished and had lost her maidenhead.

In late 1987, Jessica Hahn was the hottest commodity on the sex market. *Playboy* paid Hahn $1,000,000 for her story and it appeared in other publications at about the same time. The nude photos of this earth angel in the November 1987 issue of *Playboy* were conclusive evidence that she and "loverboy" Bakker should have made sweet music together, whether celestial or rock and roll. Bakker's downfall was Jessica's rise to stardom. Her religion paid off, possibly with some physical and mental aches and pains. Bakker also was caught with his hands in the cookie jar. He admittedly attempted to buy little Jessie's silence with $265,000 from donated church funds.

There's another facet of Jim Bakker—accusations of bisexual conduct. All this must have been a shattering disillusion to Bakker's wife Tammy and the more than 13 million devoted followers and supporters of this head of a vast multimillion-dollar television/ theme park ministry, who is now serving an eighteen-year prison sentence. It was something more than a shattering disillusion to the many thousands of Bakker's followers whom he fleeced out of their life's savings and left penniless. How could such a nice guy go so far astray? He was every bit as morally corrupt as the more recent savings and loan swindlers.

Another real shocker was in early 1988 when the superstar of religious show biz, Jimmy Swaggart, let his human instincts get him caught up in worldly pleasures. He said, the devil made him do it. At the same time Swaggart was having an immoral relationship with a prostitute, he referred to Jim Bakker as "a cancer on the Body of Christ." Oh ye, who cast the first stone— where is the integrity? Swaggart is not only deceptive, he is despicable. Perhaps, I too have been deceptive; however, my deception has only involved a handful of people, not 50,000,000 worldwide dedicated, financially supporting followers. I do believe most of the television evangelists, with the exception of one or two, are driven by unconscionable motives. They're in it for the money and the perpetuation of their own personal opulence. For the most part, they are exceptional dramatic actors. Swaggart has the cunning theatrical ability to sweat and cry at the drop of a handkerchief. He does it in almost every performance and his fans love it. They send and give him, alone, hundreds of millions. It's a strange thing, these "men of the cloth" tell you to pray to God for your needs and wants and at the same time ask you to fulfill theirs by sending money. I could be a fantastic television evangelist. I have the demeanor and an articulate speaking ability, but I have one big hang-up: a conscience.

Virtuous Exceptions

Of course, there are exceptions. My all-time favorite Protestant clergyman is Robert Harold Schuller, the West Coast counterpart of New York's Norman Vincent Peale, both of whose religious affiliation is the Dutch Reformed Church of America. In less than four years, Schuller completed the world-famous Crystal Cathedral at a staggering cost of $18,000,000, twice the original estimate due to overruns and inflation. And, upon completion, this awesome edifice was debt free. Dr. Schuller is a man who moves mountains.

Schuller is not a hell fire and brimstone preacher of the gospel. If you have ever heard or seen him on television, you know he is a suave, sophisticated, convincing motivationalist. Robert Schuller, the former Iowa farm boy, has become one of the greatest spiritual entrepreneurs of our time. I have met and talked with him on two separate occasions. One time I asked him what his thoughts were about homosexuality. Schuller's simple reply was, "God didn't intend for it to be that way." He has an overpowering, fascinating attraction and money seems to flow in his direction. He also has the inordinate capability of influencing people to recast, improve, and enrich their lives. While I was in business in Orange County, Sue and I would attend his monthly "Possibility Thinkers" luncheons at the Crystal Cathedral, and each time we would take along, as our guests, one or two of our key employees. The luncheons always featured a visiting outstanding motivational speaker. One of the guests we were most impressed with was Art Linkletter.

When I think of a truly virtuous, holy person only one name comes to mind—Mother Teresa of Calcutta. This tireless, frail, little angel of mercy, born Agnes Bojaxhiu in Yugoslavia in 1910, is known in India as "the saint of the gutters." She founded the order Missionaries of Charity, whose nuns and brothers span the globe. She has touched the lives of millions and money also flows in her direction. You may recall, in 1979 she was a recipient of the Nobel Peace Prize. Sometime after her death, Mother Teresa will undoubtedly be canonized a saint. However, the church moves slowly in matters of sainthood and this probably will not happen until well into the next century, certainly not in my lifetime.

I have vented my wrath on religion and more particularly on my religion, Catholicism. For many years the teachings of the Catholic church compounded my psychosexual dilemma with a sinful guilt syndrome. If the church is to play a significant role in the lives of modern men and women, Rome must tolerate the challenge of recognizing the realities of sex in its variable expressions and forms. Sex will be the ruination of religion unless all churches face up to it in the twentieth century. That doesn't leave us much time. Vatican reforms could stem a Catholic church revolt. The church is in such disarray on matters concerning sex, I don't believe I have anything to worry about regarding my sexuality, either in the here or in the hereafter.

10

A Look Back—Some Regrets

Writing this book has been somewhat of a nightmare. I wanted so badly to do it that it became a fervent obsession. From the bottom of my heart, I was convinced I could contribute a better understanding of the gay person to our society. Now that the ravaging AIDS crisis has put homosexuality in the limelight and an intense focus on the gay lifestyle, millions of average Americans want to know what it's all about. What is a gay? What are the factors that contribute to this sexual preference? And in view of AIDS, what does the future hold? To tell it like it is, I couldn't candy-coat the elements or issues. I believe that, to do it right, I couldn't pull any punches, even though sometimes certain revelations might be distasteful.

This book is not for gays; they know the story. It has been written for the vast number of Americans who are inquisitive and perplexed about the heterogeneous, enigmatic issue of homosexuality. I'm a gay who finds it difficult to differentiate between heterosexual love and homosexual sex—an undeniable quandary in my life. I believe my story will be perceived by straight people as a cultural revelation, rather than a self-incriminating exposé of a double life.

When I plotted the project, my number-one priority was secrecy and confidentiality. I could not let my wife know what I was doing or anyone else, for that matter. So my writing became a surreptitious undertaking. For the most part, this book was written during many business trips, which I made for an international management-consulting firm, my present employer. I had numerous think sessions with myself to refresh my memory about the many things that happened to me and the situations I have been involved in for the past thirty to forty years—things my wife will never know about. Many wives never know the shrouded inner secrets of their husband's minds.

It's awfully hard to write in the confines of the "closet." But in this "closet" I have spent untold hours of research in compiling data, research that gives this book irrefutable credibility. There is no hearsay or conjecture here. All names, places, dates, and numbers have been investigated and verified and every consequential, significant statement has been researched and documented. It has involved numerous contacts with various city, county, state, and federal government agencies, as well as newspaper librarians, church spokesmen, and others.

I didn't realize it when I started writing this book, but for a number of reasons, *Half Straight* may have a personal impact on the lives of many readers. People may start to wonder: What about my husband? Could I have a son or daughter who is part of this unconventional lifestyle? What about my dear, good friends I believe I know so well? In some people's minds, *Half Straight* may trigger uncertainty and suspicion.

There has been a multitude of books written on the subject of homosexuality. I have read many of them and you may be assured that none tell of and depict the gay culture as I have in these pages. I have tried to write this book so it would be understood in simple terms by everyone, straight and gay, and in doing so may have at times overstepped the bounds of propriety. But I felt that this approach was better than that taken by professionals in the fields of psychology and sociology, whose case histories are boring reading by most standards. To the average person they would be considered heavy folderol and gobbledygook, although they are the results of countless hours of fact-finding inquiry. Most of these books refer to the realm of homosexuality as a subculture. There is nothing "sub" about homosexuality. Within the next generation it will be as ordinary as "mom and apple pie."

Because of my close relationship with my immediate family and our conventional home life, I know a hell of a lot more about being straight than a straight person knows about being gay. Since I am some of both, I am in a unique position to comment on both lifestyles. Many men who live in the straight lifestyle are homosexual all their lives and never face up to it. They rationalize by telling themselves that their conduct is different from that of the stereotyped "swishy" homosexual and so refuse to admit they are one. They consider themselves big-hunk macho men, lacking in humanity's best-loved virtues so often found in women, such as tenderness, sensitivity, receptivity, and empathy.

Homosexuality is such an intricate mesh of behavior, emotions, and traits that it is hard to define a typical homosexual personality. A person may have none of the stereotypical behavior characteristics and still be homosexual. For a man to declare himself as a homosexual in today's society means his condemnation as a sexual loser, since a significant part of the male role is laying women. And that's where bisexuality has an advantage over homosexuality. A bisexual can play the roles that society approves of, yet savor the pleasures of both worlds. Sex for a bisexual is easier because, ordinarily, women through their natural instincts have sex only in the context of an emotional relationship, whereas men, and particularly gay men, will have sex at the blink of an eye with total strangers.

Many straight people assume that gay men relate to one

another sexually only by playing male/female roles; this idea is pure nonsense. Masculine men are attracted to masculine men. Usually, the more masculine and handsome a man is, the more masculine and handsome must be another man to interest him. Research has shown that only one out of twenty homosexuals is detectable; 95 percent of all gay people do not fit the stereotypes. To look at an individual and speculate that he or she is gay is a farcical presupposition. No one, except the men with whom I have had sex, could possibly know I'm gay, in spite of the fact that I wear Estée Lauder men's cologne from time to time.

It could be a family tragedy if my bisexuality became known, so I can't beat the drums for the gay cause. This book is my way of contributing to the cause. Undoubtedly it would be an incomprehensible shock to my family and lifelong friends if they knew I had written this book. Hopefully, in the not too distant future attitudes will change. With the slow but steady acceptance of homosexuals in our society today, there is a groundswell of gay pride. Gays, both men and women, hold responsible jobs, including management in all professions and trades. Gays are an influential factor in the voting booth. Avowed gays are being elected to powerful public offices. Homosexually oriented people who previously frequented bars, baths, and cruising areas, in order to find others like themselves, may now meet in academic discussion groups, social clubs, political assemblies, and a wide variety of religious organizations without fear of surveillance or harassment.

Nonetheless, the United States remains one of the few countries in the world where the state actively defines, regulates, and punishes adult citizens for any and all noncoital sexual activity. In some states, the government has legal jurisdiction over the human right to the use of one's own body, and its legal and social institutions may interfere in one's personal life. Yet according to credible research (Kinsey), more than a third of our country's male population has committed homosexual acts, making all those individuals criminals by our statute laws. These laws are the vestiges of outmoded religious and social mores. They stem from a fundamentalist interpretation of the Bible, which has often been used to justify all sorts of prejudice. The Bible labels all such noncoital sexual acts "sodomy," a term of infamy and disgrace. Little do the conforming bigots realize that they may have a father, mother, brother, sister, son, or daughter who falls into the same category of people they condemn. Someday they will come to the realization that being gay is no more of a sin than being black is a mark of inferiority.

Some months ago a young man of the Mormon faith appeared on a network show to let the world know he had been "cured" of his homosexuality through spiritual therapy. Homosexuality is no more curable than heterosexuality. From time to time the Catholic Church administers exorcism, as a soul-healing ministry to drive out demons from certain individuals. Nonetheless, the church has learned, in its efforts to rid priests of homosexuality, that exorcism does not work. Bisexuality is not a curable biological or mental malady. If it were, it would be like someone going into AA saying, I won't drink any more hard liquor, but I may have a beer or glass of wine now and then. If you are bisexual, to give up one means giving up both, and I don't want to live the remainder of my life in celibacy as a neuter gender in a unisex environment.

In 1973, the American Psychiatric Association removed homosexuality from psychiatry's official lexicon of mental derangements. If nothing else, this should have convinced the holier-than-thou moralists that gays are not mentally unbalanced and suffering from a character and personality disorder. The APA decision that homosexuality is no longer considered a sickness had reverberating effects on the moral issues of gay life. It added credence to the belief that homosexuality is natural and normal. That scientific decision, after years of long and laborious research and consideration probably had as much effect on gay culture as the entire thirty-five-year gay liberation movement. As a matter of fact, the APA decision was an indirect outcome of the long, bitter fight for equality and recognition by the gay liberationists. I was happy to hear of the Psychiatric Association's action since I was having a ball and didn't consider myself mentally ill because of it.

If I was destined to be one or the other, God has truly been good to me in letting me be bisexual rather than an unmixed homosexual. I suppose I could have fallen on one side of the fence or the other, but I had already known the joys of heterosexual love and sex. I'm sure I didn't know what direction I was headed when I let myself become involved in my first two homosexual encounters. I have made many mistakes in my life and there are some things I would never do again, like my long-running indiscriminate use of amyl nitrite and nitrate. Hindsight is almost always better than foresight and you just can't turn the clock back, as much as I'd like to. I'm sure I would have been much more sexually active in my youth and earlier years if I had known then what I know now. So, I expect to enjoy the next few years as a "dirty old man."

I have been around and seen and done many things in my life and undoubtedly there will be many more things to see and do in the future. My adventurous spirit has led me to ups and downs in my ambivalent life. That same spirit has created both sexual diversion and the anguishing torment I have lived with for nearly forty years. In reality, I'm proud of my strength and adeptness in coping with a preposterous enigma for two-thirds of my life.

I was born under the zodiac sign of Virgo, which gives me the dubious distinction of being a perfectionist. I suppose I really have been a picky, fastidious, persnickety guy all my life. I have long adhered to this proverb—"You don't get a second chance to make a first impression." When I was at my lowest ebb financially, physically, and mentally, if the occasion called for it, I'd dress as the chairman of the board and play the role to the hilt. Virgos are very proud people in addition to being perfectionists. My wife has always said she doesn't worry about me playing around on the side because she believes I wouldn't go to bed with another woman unless she first produced a health department certificate. Too bad that such an intelligent woman could be so naive. Sue would die if she knew my other side. There are millions of women like her, women who still don't know their husbands even after a long lifetime of marriage.

One of my sisters recently said to me, "You've got to slow down; you're not the boy you used to be." My retort was, "I have an unrestrained and unlimited energy reserve, but still there is no place in it for slowing down."

My prime and ultimate ambition is to be a millionaire. Two hundred Americans become millionaires every day and I only want to earn my share. I have several irons in the fire and a workable plan for achieving this goal. However, it can't materialize by me slowing down. My sister said, "I don't know why you want so much money; it may only bring you misery." I said, "I'd rather be miserable with it than without it. There's going to be just so much misery in our lives anyway."

I have great plans for the future and no intention of slowing down; I can't if I hope to remain physically, mentally, and sexually active. Victor Hugo said, "Forty is the old age of youth and fifty is the youth of old age." I like to think I'm still within the range of the latter. If there is any truth in the adage "Life begins at forty," I'm still in my second youth. Obviously, I didn't say my second childhood—that begins at eighty. My wife and I jog, swim, and ride bicycles together, and at age sixty-five I've got my second wind. The outlook for the future is tremendously exciting to me and there is ample time to pursue and achieve my goals and objectives.

I don't want to be like the average Joe who loses the zest

for living in middle age. A good example was one of my life-
long straight friends, who died some time ago. He was one of
the "skinny dipping" crowd when we were in high school. He
worked for a public utility for about thirty-five years, and wanted
long-range security rather than opportunity. When he was seventeen or eighteen years old, he was fired up with excitement
and enthusiasm about the future. But after coming home from
World War II, getting married, and starting to raise a family,
his zest for achieving the good life began to diminish. He became satisfied being just another number in the time clock and
eventually lost all ambition. When we were in high school, he
was an inspiration to me because of his ideals and exuberance.
In recent years he was looking forward to an early retirement.
He retired and a year later was buried as the result of a heart
attack. In terms of economic wealth, he left little to his family.

In this book I have sounded like a totally uninhibited, flamboyant, exhibitionist sex fiend. In reality, I'm a very modest, private individual and will keep my identity confidential. Outwardly, I'm the All-American family man and that's a great image.
However, on the other side of this double life, I'm a different
individual, and now you know it after reading this book. You
must also be aware that there is, indeed, a gay culture and that
homosexuality is something to be reckoned with. It has been
around since the origin of the human species and it's not going
to go away.

There are undoubtedly people who, after reading this book,
may consider it a disgusting experience. If they truly feel that
way, it nevertheless must have been a mind-boggling and en-
lightening adventure. They have been exposed to an educational insight that isn't in the curriculum of any university. People
who take exception to and disapprove of what they have read
here may be gay as well as straight. There are millions of gays
who know nothing of the gay bar and bath scene. These same
people may never have heard of "poppers," "tearooms," "glory

holes," "dildos," "cock rings," and the Metropolitan Community Church. They live in the hinterlands and byways of our country, as well as the big cities and suburban areas. I only hope what I have written here will give them confidence and inspire them to face the future with courage, knowing there are many millions like them throughout the world.

I have a viable, plausible plan to share the proceeds from the publishing of this book with my wife and at the same time never let her know the book exists. However, first of all, 10 percent off the top goes to God (my favorite religious charity). I couldn't have accomplished this project without Him; He was with me all the way. I realized from the start it would take unmitigated guts, but something kept urging me on, in spite of the secretive handicaps I worked under. All legal bases will be covered and all IRS and other taxes will be paid. If someone were successful in piercing my veil of secrecy, I would reveal my identity before I would fall prey to blackmail or extortion.

What would I do if I had it to do all over again? That's hard to say. I've been bisexual two-thirds of my life and even though I'm somewhat of a social loner, I have for many years been a sexual extrovert, driven by a passionate lust for sex in any form. Bisexuality has added an exhilarating dimension to my life, one that straight people can't seem to comprehend. I do know now that my psychosexual biology and its frustrations have affected my very nature, causing an emotional impact on the ones I truly love so much, even though they don't know the basis of my conduct. It's becoming a gut-wrenching realization that my mean temperament and hostile demeanor, at times, with my family for many long years may have eroded into repulsive resentment; I keep getting the vibes.

The most rueful of all my regrets has been my powerless inability to wholeheartedly cope with my sex-oriented psychological complexities. I know there have been times my relationship and behavior with my family have bordered on tyrannical, despite my deep-rooted love for my wife and son and daughter. And then there are "The Days of Wine and Roses." Sue has been the long-suffering victim of not just one but two monkeys on my back. Now, I believe I have mellowed with age and only wish I could turn the clock back so it could have been a full lifetime of cool temper, enduring love, unwavering devotion, and outgoing affection for the one who means the most to me—my wife.

Psychologists tell us this is the age of multiple personalities. Obviously, I have a dual sexual personalty, but my family and closest friends know of only one. If I had known I were gay at age eighteen or nineteen, I'm sure I wouldn't have gotten married. In that case I may have turned out to be homosexual rather than bisexual. But, as I think about that, it would have deprived me of some of life's greatest joys—my dear wife, my cherished daughter and son, and in more recent years our son-in-law and beloved grandkids. All these have to be the greatest blessings in anyone's life. Nonetheless, I haven't had any real peace of mind since the day of my first gay encounter, although it was by happenstance. The emotional aspects of this autobiography, in many ways, tell a sad story, although I have attempted to inject a little humor along the way. Overtly, my psychobiology has made a hell of a mess of my life. On the other hand, there are times I think the fulfillment has outweighed any conforming. Obviously I am a confused, complex heterogeneous individual—a mix of good and bad, hopefully more of the former.

I have taken a bold and hazardous gamble by "spilling my guts" and revealing my experiences with gay culture, a gamble that could mean my ruination if my identity became known. To some it may be critiqued as a sordid disclosure, but it's simply a fact of life. Intelligent, well-adjusted people can take this in stride. We're in the countdown to the end of the twentieth century and I believe most people now have a compelling, searching curiosity about what's actually taking place in our society. I have told my personal story without reservation and to my knowledge such an all-inclusive saga of a bisexual life has never been published with such candor and with the mixed emotions I have expressed here.

Epilogue

Undoubtedly, this true story has been a relevation to most straight readers. After reading this book, those who were in the dark on this subject can no longer be either ignorant or naive.

It should now be apparent that we gays are ordinary people who, by fate, have become what we are. We have heartfelt human feelings, just as all of God's mortal beings. We are not bizarre dregs of society because of our sexual orientation, and most of us don't deserve being targets of the homophobia syndrome. It's only a small minority of the gay population that attracts distasteful, embarrassing attention.

It is my sincere hope that the readers of this book will have a new compassion for and be more tolerant of their friends, neighbors, associates, and loved ones who like me show signs of personality flaws—whether it be arrogance, cynicism, egotism, or a temperamental disposition. The unsuspected, underlying cause of their behavior may be homosexuality. Before you condemn us, think of the old adage: There but for the grace of God go I.

THE AUTHOR